Age
Strong

A WOMAN'S GUIDE TO FEELING ATHLETIC AND FIT AFTER 40

Rachel Cosgrove

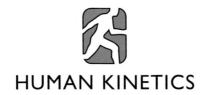

HUMAN KINETICS

Library of Congress Cataloging-in-Publication Data

Names: Cosgrove, Rachel, author.
Title: Age strong : a woman's guide to feeling athletic and fit after 40 /
  Rachel Cosgrove.
Other titles: Woman's guide to feeling athletic and fit after forty
Description: First edition. | Champaign, IL : Human Kinetics, [2024] |
  Includes bibliographical references.
Identifiers: LCCN 2023049904 (print) | LCCN 2023049905 (ebook) | ISBN
  9781718220775 (print : alk. paper) | ISBN 9781718220782 (epub) | ISBN
  9781718220799 (pdf)
Subjects: LCSH: Weight training for women. | Exercise for women. | Physical
  fitness for women. | Muscle strength--Training. | Weight training. |
  Women--Health and hygiene. | Women--Nutrition. | Exercise for
  middle-aged persons. | BISAC: HEALTH & FITNESS / Exercise / Strength
  Training | HEALTH & FITNESS / Women's Health
Classification: LCC GV546.6.W64 C67 2024 (print) | LCC GV546.6.W64
  (ebook) | DDC 613.7/1082--dc23/eng/20231201
LC record available at https://lccn.loc.gov/2023049904
LC ebook record available at https://lccn.loc.gov/2023049905

ISBN: 978-1-7182-2077-5 (print)

This publication is written and published to provide accurate and authoritative information relevant to the subject matter presented. It is published and sold with the understanding that the author and publisher are not engaged in rendering legal, medical, or other professional services by reason of their authorship or publication of this work. If medical or other expert assistance is required, the services of a competent professional person should be sought.

The web addresses cited in this text were current as of September 2023, unless otherwise noted.

Senior Acquisitions Editor: Michelle Earle; **Senior Developmental Editor:** Cynthia McEntire; **Managing Editor:** Shawn Donnelly; **Copyeditor:** Michelle Horn; **Permissions Manager:** Laurel Mitchell; **Senior Graphic Designer:** Joe Buck; **Cover Designer:** Keri Evans; **Cover Design Specialist:** Susan Rothermel Allen; **Photograph (cover):** © Human Kinetics; **Photographs (interior):** © Human Kinetics, unless otherwise noted; **Photo Production Specialist:** Amy M. Rose; **Photo Production Manager:** Jason Allen; **Senior Art Manager:** Kelly Hendren; **Illustrations:** © Human Kinetics, unless otherwise noted; **Printer:** Versa Press

We thank Results Fitness in Newhall, California, for assistance in providing the location for the photo shoot for this book.

Human Kinetics books are available at special discounts for bulk purchase. Special editions or book excerpts can also be created to specification. For details, contact the Special Sales Manager at Human Kinetics.

Printed in the United States of America

10 9 8 7 6 5 4 3 2 1

The paper in this book is certified under a sustainable forestry program.

Human Kinetics
1607 N. Market Street
Champaign, IL 61820
USA

United States and International
Website: **US.HumanKinetics.com**
Email: info@hkusa.com
Phone: 1-800-747-4457

Canada
Website: **Canada.HumanKinetics.com**
Email: info@hkcanada.com

E9062

This book is dedicated to all the women who have joined Results Fitness over the years, trusting us to help them reach their peak health and fitness in their 40s, 50s, 60s, and beyond. Thank you for being an example of aging strong to inspire every reader of this book.

CONTENTS

PART I   STRENGTH TRAINING IN YOUR 40S AND BEYOND

PART II   PREPARE FOR POSITIVE CHANGE

PART III   THE EXERCISES

PART IV   THE AGE STRONG PROGRAM

EXERCISE FINDER

Warm-Up Exercises

Core Exercises

Upper-Body Exercises

Lower-Body Exercises

Power Development, Finishers, and Metabolic Intervals

FOREWORD
BY JILL COLEMAN

Have you ever had the experience of seeing someone walk into a room, and the energy completely changes? The room becomes charged with a sense of power and poise, and the person you're watching commands the attention of others without having to say a word? That is exactly how I felt the first time I saw Rachel speak on stage.

The first time I met my mentor Rachel Cosgrove was at a fitness business event. She was presenting and, at the time, I was a very new online fitness coach and painfully insecure. In my 20s, I tried my hand at fitness modeling and figure competitions. This type of physique-fixation can encourage things such as disordered eating, body dysmorphia, self-esteem issues, and general body self-consciousness. I was young and wanted to see how far I could push myself and my body and, in doing so, ended up yo-yo dieting for years, losing and gaining the same 10 to 20 pounds multiple times per year, never feeling lean enough, fit enough, or good enough. In my naiveté, I'd associated thinness and smallness with good-enough-ness. The ironic part was, the skinnier I got, the more insecure I became.

Enter Rachel. She was a few years my senior but was also a successful gym owner, businesswoman, author, and speaker. She had the exact type of success I wanted (hence why she eventually became my mentor). But she wasn't chasing skinny. She was powerful, confident, well-spoken, and clearly self-possessed while also being a fit, athletic woman in her 40s.

Rachel's example set in motion a complete paradigm shift for me. Here was someone who wasn't trying to get smaller but commanded a room, had massive success, and clearly owned all of it. I wanted that, too.

In 2012, when I first worked with Rachel, I was dieting for a speaking gig. The nonstop excessive cardio and calorie-cutting was a full-time job, and I remember Rachel telling me that if I wanted to speak on more stages and *really* do this business thing—have massive success—I needed to own my power. And the constant dieting was stealing it. How could I serve the masses when all I focused on was myself and my need to look a certain way? Rachel helped me see that making a massive impact can't be about me. It has to be about others.

From then on, I simply owned it. I booked speeches and held workshops and didn't think twice about needing to be skinnier or smaller. I focused my time in the gym on weight-training, lifting heavier, and over the years felt my power come back. Ironically, the physique I've built is one I love so much more than the skinny, scared kid I once was.

At 42 years old now, I can say that I am proud of the body I've built through weights and the success I've had because of Rachel's example. I credit Rachel with not only helping me change how I view the intersection of business, fitness, power, and femininity, but for being a pioneer in our space in the early days of internet coaching and certainly one of the first females blazing a trail for the rest of us.

I imagine it's hard to go first, but Rachel has always led from the front, and continues to inspire the newest generation of fit pros, as well as the general population. I can't think of someone more well-suited to lead the over-40 female crowd to becoming stronger, fitter, and more athletic, yes, even in the second half of life. This book is a gift, and I can't wait to see the millions of lives changed as a result.

Thank you, Rachel. Love you, lady. Forever grateful.

Xo, Jill (aka JillFit)

INTRODUCTION

"Being in your 60s now looks a lot different than it used to," said a client as she flexed her 60-year-old biceps while wearing a tank top that she never would have felt confident in during her 40s. Heck yes, it does! Women aren't afraid to have muscles, be strong, and make time for themselves. Throughout this book, you will learn about making the most of your 40s, 50s, 60s, 70s, and beyond.

You want to live longer and test the odds? Have more personal power in determining your health from how you move to how you feel and enjoy life? Turning another year older, such as the big 5-0, can be frightening and motivating, but also a turning point. For women who strength train, it can also lead to the realization that they are in the best shape of their lives and doing things they never thought possible, despite getting older! Many of my clients at Results Fitness are reaching their peak health and fitness in their 50s and even 60s.

At Results Fitness, women in their 40s to 70s are lifting weights at least twice a week like their lives depend on it, because they do. These women have learned that being strong means being healthy. They have learned that their mood and stress levels are better after a heavy lifting session. They have seen themselves progress every year, first able to do 5 push-ups, now 6 push-ups, now 10 push-ups, now 15 push-ups, now with a weight on their back! The progress never stops! They get stronger, fitter, and healthier every year. They see their blood panels and bone density improve when others start seeing themselves at risk for osteoporosis. It's common for my clients' doctors to ask what they are doing!

Personally, as I turned 40, I couldn't motivate myself to step up my training and dial in my nutrition to feel my best. I looked and felt "good enough." I don't get on the scale much, so it wasn't until my annual physical in August 2016 that I realized I had gained weight every year for the last six years. It was gradual, 2 or 3 pounds (about 1 kg) a year, and I was now, at 41 years old, 15 pounds (7 kg) heavier than I was at 35 years old. Maybe I had gained muscle? I jumped on our Inbody Body Composition Analyzer to find out.

Even more disturbing than the weight gain was the fact that I had reached an unhealthy 30 percent body fat. How did this happen? This trend cannot continue! I refused to become a statistic of the "it's harder to stay in shape as you get older" mentality.

I'm a fitness expert, and I pride myself on leading by example. Plus, I feel better when I'm fit. I set the goal to be in the best shape of my life by the time I turned 50. I see clients rocking 50 years old and beyond all the time! I was ready to turn this around. I want to be healthy and fit as I age.

Spotlight on Donna Lee

Member since 2011

How old were you when you started strength training, and how old are you now?

I was 48 years old when I started at Results Fitness, but I had been lifting light weights before that as a step aerobics instructor. I'm now 60 years young.

Why did you decide to make strength training a priority?

With a background as an endurance athlete, running was always my go-to, along with being a softball coach and teaching PE and aerobics classes. I joined Results Fitness, initially sticking to their group classes and doing the metabolic interval workouts. I started lifting in their group strength training workouts and was quickly lifting the heaviest kettlebell and heaviest sandbag, so I needed more. At that point, I moved from only doing group classes to working with a coach and learning more about challenging myself with strength training, where I saw dramatically faster results as I got stronger, leaner, and fitter. The heavier I lifted, the better I felt. Having a customized strength training program made a big difference for me.

What was your experience going through perimenopause and menopause?

I was 52 years old, and overall, it really didn't affect me like I know it does some women. I remember having some hot flashes, and a year later my period stopped. I really didn't notice any changes in my body, which may have been because at the same time I had embraced a structured serious strength training program, so I was making more progress with my fitness than I had in a while.

What results did you get by prioritizing strength training?

My body feels so much better now than it did when I was in my 40s. The results came dramatically quicker by prioritizing strength training than with cardio/aerobic classes. When I was in my 40s, I never would have worn a tank top. Now, in my 60s, I'm always wearing a tank top. I'm so much more confident. I remember my mom being 60 and how different my 60s are from my mom's 60s. I'm still gaining muscle and strength at 60, and it's the best feeling ever. Since getting serious with my strength training, I've set and reached several goals and continue to keep setting new goals. I compete in the Tactical Strength Challenge (a strength challenge of deadlifts, snatches, and pull-ups) every year, challenging myself to do more than the year before; I competed in a bikini competition; I did a Spartan obstacle course race; and I've run three marathons. I also love seeing all the women in the gym lifting weights and getting stronger no matter their age.

How many days a week do you lift weights?

I've been in a routine of four days a week of strength training for the last five years religiously.

What have you found to work for your nutrition goals?

I am a schoolteacher. I have a routine of three meals a day and usually two snacks of something quick on the go between periods, like a handful of nuts. I eat dinner pretty early at five p.m., and then I don't eat for the rest of the night. I work out every morning fueled by half a power bar and then I eat a big, high-protein breakfast, usually eggs, after my workout. And I double up on my postworkout protein with a recovery shake. I drink 100 ounces of water a day and make sure to get protein at every meal. I eat lots of fish, chicken, and ground turkey. I love ground turkey.

What do you recommend to someone who is in their 40s wanting to age strong?

Carve out some "me" time *now*. That's why I started running initially. It's so important to find a time for you. Connect with a community and get a group of friends to have an outlet. In your 40s, the people you surround yourself with will make a big difference. Getting input from others who are in a similar place to you is so important. Being around all the women in the gym strength training, I see I'm not the only one in my 60s getting strong, fit, and healthy. We support each other and cheer each other on. We all need that.

I recognized that I had fallen into some nutritional habits over the years, not caring as much, eating what I wanted when I wanted, probably having a few too many splurges that were adding up, and, yes, making excuses along with not having a focused goal in the gym. I do much better with a goal!

Since I started checking my progress, my body composition changed slowly in recent years. I dropped 15 pounds (7 kg) of fat in 17 months while gaining 3 pounds (1 kg) of muscle! I didn't do anything extreme. In fact, wine and pizza are a weekly occurrence. I've made slow, steady progress in the right direction.

Now at 48 years old, I've maintained my body composition while learning new skills and competing in a new sport, obstacle course racing, as an age-group competitor. This gave me a goal and focus for my training. We'll talk more about this in the chapter on goal setting. Most importantly I'm stronger and healthier than I have been in a while!

It's easy to slide gradually as we age, losing muscle, gaining fat, decreasing our ability to do things, and getting out of touch with the athlete within. As we enter our 40s, we hit a crossroads when we can either take control and work to gain strength and fitness and improve our health, or we'll start to lose muscle and bone mass and become more prone to injury and disease.

Writing this book is partly selfish as I looked through all the research studies surrounding topics of menopause and aging while also spending a lot of time interviewing dozens of clients at Results Fitness who started working out in their 40s right through to now, when they are in their 60s and even 70s. The gym has been open 23 years, so I have access to a large pool of women who have trained right through the transition and are now on the other side of menopause and able to share their experiences. I searched for the commonalities among clients—strength training, sleep, stress relief, and nutrition—to land on what seems to be the answer to aging strong. Results Fitness is a real-world research and development laboratory. I don't know too many research studies done over 23 years following more than 20 women from their 40s to their 60s. In this book, you'll learn the findings and get to know some of these women.

Many of these women started as completely sedentary as they approached their 40s, having lost touch with being an athlete or never knowing that they could be an athlete. I'll be sharing stories of women from their 40s to their 70s who you'll realize are doing so much more than they would have been if they had never started to lift weights.

One client joined Results Fitness at 57 years old and is now 68 years old (you'd *never* know). As she bent over to touch her toes after swinging a kettlebell, she said, "I was never athletic growing up, so now that I've discovered the athlete I am, this is my childhood!" She and her husband regularly hike difficult mountain ranges as a personal challenge. She now realizes there are no limits as she approaches her 70s!

If you saw one of these women, you'd ask yourself what sport she plays or what kind of athlete she is. Most important, they are totally confident with their bodies and feel good about themselves, never feeling like "It's too late" or "I'm too old." They are empowered, fit, and strong in their 40s and beyond.

What you might not be able to tell is that they are in their 40s or 50s or 60s. What do they know that you don't know?

They know how to lift weights properly, and it's part of their weekly routine at least twice a week. They know how to fuel their bodies like athletes with enough protein and veggies. They know how to recover with eight hours of sleep a night. They know they can set a goal to accomplish something new because it's not too late. They know they have control over looking and feeling exactly like they want, never using age as an excuse again.

Throughout the years, I noticed that many women who decide to start an exercise routine as they approach their 40s lift weights that are too light, barely breaking a sweat, unaware of their strength and what it will take to build muscle. Or they're afraid to even touch the weights in fear of hulk-like muscles popping up on their body or falling into the "I'm older and therefore weaker" stereotype.

These same women won't think twice about doing three cardio classes in a row, sweating it out on their Peloton, and spending countless hours walking. With this effort, these women don't understand why their bodies look and feel exactly the same as they did six months ago and why it's getting harder and harder to make any progress. They start to have joints that ache and pain in places they didn't before.

Don't get me wrong, walking every day is important and needs to be a part of the recipe for aging strong. The problem is that it is not going to build muscle and strength. When talking to women in their 40s about their exercise routines, I've heard many tell me, "I walk." Period. That's the entire exercise routine.

They have been misinformed and need help, which is why I'm so passionate about writing this book! If walking is the only exercise you do, you are setting yourself up to have less muscle and therefore less strength and independence along with more injuries and a slower metabolism as you age. Some of these women may not know what else to do or how to lift weights properly to get strong. I also realize the weight training floor can be very intimidating.

Men have always had the perspective that they can do it and can always do more, getting stronger, bigger, faster, leaner, etc. On the other hand, women have often heard they can't do anything—they can't do push-ups or chin-ups, and they can't lift heavy. It all started when the generation now turning 40 was young and told to do girl push-ups, the implication being that their gender made them weaker than boys.

Most women don't do anything other than a "girl push-up" for the rest of their lives, thinking, "I am a girl; I can't do a real push-up!" Go to any women's only section of a gym, and you'll see pink dumbbells probably up to 15 pounds (7 kg). There is nothing there to challenge a woman to work out hard. It's common for a woman to feel intimidated in the gym because of the presence of a man, or she might feel pressured give up a machine or a bench because a man is waiting for it. So much of it is confidence and attitude! Self-esteem and confidence are all part of the package that go along with my philosophies on how a woman needs to approach her workouts in the gym as she gets older. When asking our clients what strength training has given them, almost all of them say confidence, along with a long list of other benefits. That confidence is one of the most important benefits of getting strong: confidence to be able to do the things you want to do, confidence to wear what you want to wear, confidence to say "yes" to life experiences.

This book is written to convince you that if you're a woman over 40, lifting weights—and not just the light pink ones—will give you the confidence and empowerment to be active as you age. Heading into your 40s or later, if you haven't embraced weight training as a necessary part of your routine, it's time to start lifting weights. It's time to start feeling confident when approaching a squat rack or setting up your own home gym with what you need, including a squat rack, barbells, and weight plates! Make it a setup any man would be jealous of. The gym is our place as much as any man's! I'm excited to introduce you to what it can do for you.

Throughout this book, I'll back up my philosophies with scientific evidence and powerful real-world examples from actual clients who have seen the benefits and my own experiences. Nothing is more motivating than to read a real-world story of someone you can connect with who was once where you are now and can show you the path they took to look and feel their best as they embraced aging. You'll also find a 16-week program that provides the exact plan to follow to start making strength training a priority, which is step one to aging strong, along with a whole chapter on living the lifestyle, including nutrition, recovery, sleep, and all the important stuff to age strong!

PART I

STRENGTH TRAINING IN YOUR 40S AND BEYOND

CHAPTER 1

WHY STRENGTH TRAIN?

You can turn 40, 50, 60, or older and still get functionally younger and stronger the next 10, 20, 30 years, or more. Strength training is the most effective way for women over 40 to stay young, fit, and strong to enjoy life year after year as they age. Unfortunately, it is too common to see women back off from doing serious workouts as they age and regress to walking as their only exercise. "I take my dog on long walks every night," one woman told me as she complained about gaining weight through menopause. Long walks are great, but shifting to prioritize lifting heavy weights is what will make the biggest difference for women in this time of their lives.

The sooner you start strength training, the better, so start now. In fact, one thing I hear from so many clients in their 60s is, "I wish I would have started serious strength training earlier." I have been coaching women in their 40s, 50s, and 60s for more than 20 years at Results Fitness with a large group of clients in the 60+ category. In fact, we have a large group of women over 60 who gather every month to support each other on their strength journeys, some who have taken up competitive powerlifting and others who compete in various sports at the National Senior Games. They call themselves the Glamourous Grannies (GGs), and all regularly strength train two or three days a week to stay young.

One of the GGs experienced joint pain associated with her job in her 40s and 50s. Realizing she was having trouble carrying her first grandchild while climbing the stairs, she realized, "This is not me!" She joined Results Fitness in her 50s. She remembers one of her first exercises was stepping onto a very low step. She thought, "This isn't going to do anything." As time went on and she progressed, she got stronger and was able to step onto a taller step with no knee pain. She went from having to ask for help at the grocery store to lift a case of water or a box at home to eventually being able to deadlift 205 pounds (93 kg) and asking others if she could help them with their cases of water. She actively helps with her grandkids and feels more confident in her abilities at age 73 than she was in her 50s.

No matter your age, you can achieve amazing results in your health and lifestyle by improving your fitness level, increasing your physical strength and endurance, and improving your aerobic capacity. Even people in their 80s who start lifting weights can get stronger with each workout. It's never too late to start. The best day to start was 20 years ago, but the second-best day to start is right now!

Let's look at some reasons why making strength training a priority is crucial to enjoying life to the fullest beyond 40 years old.

STRENGTH TRAINING INCREASES LONGEVITY

Want to be around longer to experience more in life? See your grandkids get married, be a part of your great-grandkids lives, and be in more family pictures and memories, leaving your legacy with those important to you? The *Journal of the American Heart Association* published a study in 2017 that concluded "a moderate amount of time spent strength training seemed beneficial for longevity independent of aerobic activity" (Kamada et al. 2017). Longevity is only as good as your quality of life. The stronger and fitter you are as you age, the more you'll be ready to jump in and experience.

The GG I mentioned earlier told me a story about how her family, including seven grandchildren, decided at the last minute to play volleyball in the park and invited Grandma and Grandpa to come. Did they sit on the sidelines and watch the kids play? Nope. They jumped into play alongside the family. As you age, do you want to be on the sidelines or in the game of life? Making strength training a priority will keep you ready to jump into the arena and participate. If you've never been an athlete, that's okay, too. You might find your inner athlete as you gain confidence in your strength and fitness. It makes longevity much more interesting when you can participate in all you missed out on or said no to before you discovered your newfound strength and fitness.

STRENGTH TRAINING IMPROVES YOUR ODDS OF AVOIDING AND OVERCOMING INJURY AND DISEASE

We all fear spending our later years sick, frail, and unable to enjoy life. In *Younger Next Year*, author Chris Crowley explains that more than 50 percent of illnesses and injuries in the last third of life can be eliminated by starting a fitness program (Crowley and Lodge 2004). According to the Centers for Disease Control (CDC), among the top causes of injury and death in older Americans are falling, heart disease, and cancer (Xu et al. 2022).

By maintaining a healthy and active lifestyle, you can keep your strength and balance to avoid falls, dodge chronic illnesses including heart disease and many cancers, and reduce your risk of conditions such as arthritis, diabetes, and even Alzheimer's.

Most of the clients in my gym who have trained from their 40s through their 60s have avoided being put on any medications. At all.

Arthritis is the nation's number one cause of disability, with 29.3 percent of people aged 45 to 64 years and 49.6 percent of people aged 65 year or older reporting doctor-diagnosed arthritis (CDC 2021). I suspect that more people have arthritis, with many people over 40 complaining of some kind of joint pain at some point. Arthritis refers to joint pain or joint disease, and there are more than 100 types.

Research shows that strength training is extremely beneficial for people with arthritis. Strength training helps support and protect joints by strengthening the muscles around them. By improving the strength around each joint, you can ease pain and reduce the stiffness and swelling caused by arthritis (Hurkmans et al. 2009). If there's one magic bullet to combating arthritis, it's lifting weights. I have a client who turned 70 and has been training with me since she was 47. She mentioned that everyone she knows is suffering from arthritis except her. She's had a little bit in her hands but is so thankful she really hasn't been struck with the same debilitating pain that so many of her friends in the same age group who don't strength train have been complaining about.

Women tend to be hypermobile at both the knee and hip joints and need more stability to prevent injuries. Women have a higher incidence than men of anterior cruciate ligament (ACL) tears of the knee—3.5 times greater incidence in basketball and 2.8 times greater in soccer—according to a study published in the *Journal of Orthopedics* (The Female ACL 2016). In addition, women experience a higher incidence of injuries to the hip joint; hip dysplasia and labral tears are reported more often in females than males (Groh and Herrera 2009). A strength training program can decrease the risk of both ACL and hip injuries by improving stability. The only way to create more stability is to develop strength. Improving your hip strength and mobility also can decrease back pain, which is experienced by 80 percent of adults at some point in their lives (Taylor et al. 2022).

Evidence suggests that rupture of the Achilles tendon, which is much more common in people ages 30 to 46, can also be avoided or treated without surgery by emphasizing range-of-motion exercises and weight-bearing activities early in life (Sheth et al. 2017).

Spotlight on Jan Broneer

Member since 2008

How old were you when you started strength training, and how old are you now?

I was 59 years old when I started at Results Fitness, and I just turned 73 years old.

Why did you decide to start making strength training a priority?

After being active my whole life as a collegiate-level basketball player on one of the first women's basketball teams at UCLA and then having a career as a PE teacher, where I shared my passion for athletics with others, at 57 years old, my body no longer felt like an athlete. I had been a member of a gym my whole life, consistently working out and doing what I could. Working out was non-negotiable for me. I knew I had to do it for my mental health as much as physical health. I was a member of various gyms, and I'd used seated machines where I'd guess on the weights. I realize now that I wasn't challenging myself to actually get stronger.

I had a back injury that had kept me from doing much activity at all for eight years. I couldn't even be on my feet for very long before the pain was too much. Eventually my knees started to give from being bent so much to relieve my back. Not being able to bend them led to spasms in my back, wearing a T-brace to get through the day, and eventually the end of my career as a PE teacher. I transitioned to serve as a dean at the school for five years, then retired because of physical reasons: three or four different falls, tripping, slipping, and finally a chair fell out from under me. Here I was, a high-level competitive athlete being forced to retire because I wasn't physically able to do the job.

I thought to myself, "Is it inevitable to feel this way now that I am in my 50s?" My big turning point was realizing I couldn't hold my eight-pound baby grandchild while carrying her upstairs. At that point, I decided to get help hiring a professional fitness coach and joining Results Fitness to help me figure out how to be active with a bad back and bad knees to end the downward cycle I was in.

What was your experience going through perimenopause and menopause?

I think because I was active, I didn't experience dramatic symptoms going through menopause. I never knew there was such a thing as perimenopause until recently. My only recollections of actual menopause are some hot flashes, which were tolerable. I never sought a doctor's care or needed medication of any kind for this relative annoyance. I also never realized how lucky I must have been when I hear other women's horror stories and can only attribute it to the fact that I have always been consistent with my workouts and did my best to take care of myself.

What results did you get by prioritizing strength training?

I am more confident now at 73 than I was at 59. I don't think twice about bending, reaching, or lifting anything. It's given me independence. I used to have to ask for help at the grocery store, and now I offer to help people. I took for granted everything I could do before I was injured, and now I appreciate it that much more.

Most importantly, I can be there for my grandkids, taking them to appointments and joining into their sports and am ready to jump in instead of sitting on the sidelines of life.

I feel strong and like an athlete again. I can now deadlift 205 pounds (93 kg)! I participate in competitive sports again as an athlete in Masters Track & Field, where I won a silver medal; I've competed in powerlifting; and I've completed a triathlon, a mud run, and a Spartan Race. Jan the athlete is back, and it feels like I have back a piece of who I am!

My goal now is longevity. I'm going to be here longer if I keep doing what I'm doing. Part of my motivation is seeing my mom, who is 95 years old, and what a struggle her last 20 years have been. She is a recovering alcoholic, and I never drank and knew early I wanted to do something different. My mom was always very focused on how she looked. Skinny was important, not being strong. She'd go to any measure to accomplish that, from starving herself to buying every inner thigh machine and fat burner. Seeing her so weak and frail is a good reminder of why strength training and building muscle is so important as we age. She started using a walker when she was around the age I am now! This gives me my why to be as strong as I can and focus on what I can do instead of what I look like to not spend my 80s and 90s the way she is.

The idea of being able to feel good about my body and to do things is what motivates me. Age is truly just a number. I have friends my same age who are unable to do the things I do. It's a choice I make every day to work out and make the effort to stay strong, fit, and able. Showing up to a family volleyball game in the park, do you want to sit on the sidelines or be on the court playing? I want to be on the court playing! A couple years ago I decided to get back into softball and showed up at a pick-up softball game to join in.

My goal for ages 75 to 95 is to remain upright, being able to walk under my own power without a walker. In addition, the social aspect of going to the gym where now some of my best friends are has become an unexpected additional benefit. Connecting with other women in my age group who also prioritize exercise, nutrition, and their health makes such a difference, and I know it helps keep me young.

I consider my workout as my job. When I can't go, I feel out of sorts.

How many days a week do you lift weights?

I work out every day, doing strength training three or four days a week.

What have you found to work for your nutrition?

With nutrition, my goal is immunity and longevity. I currently don't take any pills or medication, and I want to keep it that way. I have never been big on taking supplements either because I really don't like to take pills. I do take vitamin D every day. I do my best to eat enough protein, along with fruits and vegetables throughout the day. I always get my postworkout recovery shake, and do my best to fuel my body with what it needs.

What do you recommend to someone who is in their 40s wanting to age strong?

It's okay to be selfish. Set boundaries to take care of yourself. Having strength physically will give you the mental strength you need in life.

If you do require surgery or medical treatment, such as hip surgery or ACL repair, because of disease or injury, the stronger and more fit you are, the better your recovery and ability to overcome and maintain quality of life. As American fitness coach Mark Rippetoe said, "Strong people are harder to kill, and more useful in general." Even after being diagnosed with cancer and starting treatment, a stronger, healthier, and fitter body will get you through the treatment more likely to survive for many years. Train to be prepared for anything.

STRENGTH TRAINING INCREASES BONE MASS AND REDUCES THE RISK OF OSTEOPOROSIS AND OSTEOPENIA

Research suggests that women can reverse bone loss through strength training (Hoke et al. 2020). A 2018 article published in *Endocrinology and Metabolism* showed resistance exercise was highly beneficial for the preservation of bone and muscle mass as women age (Hong and Kim 2018). The women at the gym who have trained with me during their 40s to 60s have completely avoided osteoporosis, despite many of them having mothers who had severe osteoporosis. In fact, quite a few clients have reversed their risk from medium risk to low risk. For example, one client had her bone mass tested when she was 41 and was told she was at medium risk for osteopenia. She joined Results Fitness and trained for a year. She went from 110 pounds (50 kg) at 28 percent body fat to 121 pounds (55 kg) at 18 percent body fat. Her body scan showed that the weight she gained was made up of both muscle and bone, and she was now at low risk for osteoporosis and osteopenia. That's aging strong!

Some key factors to improve bone mass that need to be included as part of your training are weight-bearing activities using linear or undulating periodization, progressive overload, higher-intensity training, and compound movements. You'll learn more about these techniques in the program presented in chapter 13.

STRENGTH TRAINING INCREASES METABOLISM AND REDUCES BODY FAT

As women go through perimenopause and menopause, it can be difficult to maintain their preferred body composition. On average, during the transition, women can gain 10 to 15 pounds (5 to 7 kg) of fat, usually distributed on the belly as hormones change. Some women become insulin resistant (Monash University 2023). It's not uncommon to hear women going through this time in their life say, "I've never had a belly before. Where did this come from?"

A study in the *Journal of Strength and Conditioning* published in January 2021 compared the effects of resistance training on body fat percentage and blood biomarkers in untrained women (Cunha et al. 2021). Sixty-five women more than 60 years old were assigned to one of three groups: low volume, high volume, or control. Both the low-volume and high-volume groups performed resistance training for 12 weeks. The low-volume group performed 1 set of 8 exercises for 10 to 15 repetitions, and the high-volume group performed 3 sets. The study concluded that high-volume resistance training was the most effective strategy to reduce body fat and trunk fat and improve biomarkers in older women. The high-volume group lost almost 4 percent more body fat than the low-volume group and over 6 percent trunk fat.

The programs in this book will progress you to three sets over each phase. Do all the sets to get the best results.

Perimenopause may be the best time to take advantage of the benefits of strength training, as shown in a study in the journal *Menopause* in 2022 (Gould et al. 2022). In this study, researchers evaluated the body composition of 72 women ages 35 to 60 and found that during perimenopause, the women experienced body composition changes that included losing muscle, increasing body fat percentage, and decreasing metabolism. The study concluded that perimenopause may be the most important time for lifestyle intervention.

By lifting weights and stressing your muscles, you will increase your lean mass. The effectiveness of resistance training to improve muscular strength was confirmed in healthy older adults (Borde, Hortobagyi, and Granacher 2015). Since lean mass (muscle tissue) burns fat, you can burn more fat even at rest. The right strength training routine will give your body a metabolism boost and create an afterburn effect. Combining this with a moderate amount of cardiovascular activity will turn your body into a fat burning, athletic machine. Too much cardio at this time of life may work against you because you will eventually begin to use your hard-earned lean muscle tissue for energy, which is NOT the desired goal. Don't be afraid to lift heavy to build metabolism, boosting muscle mass to age strong.

STRENGTH TRAINING IMPROVES AEROBIC CAPACITY AND ENDURANCE

If you are an endurance athlete or enjoy going for a regular run or walk, you'll be even better at it if you lift weights. Many endurance athletes peak in their 30s or 40s. Being stronger helps you to be more efficient, improving your power and strength with every step, according to a study published in the *Scandinavian Journal of Medical Science in Sports* (Hoff, Gran, and Helgerud 2002).

A client, who is now 62, found this to be true. She started running in college and excelled on the collegiate track team. Realizing she had a talent and a passion for running, being part of a team gave her a purpose. She eventually added in some strength training with basic exercises such as crunches and push-ups to complement her number one priority of running. It wasn't until she was in her 40s that she started her first structured serious strength training program, lifting weights at Results Fitness. Before she started lifting, she noticed that her body and particularly her belly were changing in ways she didn't like. Starting a consistent lifting program really helped to combat the "menopause belly" and helped her get through menopause with very few symptoms. Strength training made her stronger, and she noticed her speed increase as she felt more powerful with her running. She decided to compete in longer distances because she was feeling stronger and completed her first marathon in her 50s. While training for the marathon, she kept strength training a priority twice a week, knowing how important it was for her running performance. She found that by running less and making room in her schedule for strength training, she was getting faster! Faster with less running? Yes! Being strong gave her the confidence to push her downhill speed knowing her joints could handle it, and she was able to achieve new personal records on her 5K times. In a routine that she sees as non-negotiable because it works, she's now up to strength training three days a week. She has become certified as a personal trainer and coaches at Results Fitness. She did her first Spartan obstacle course race at 61 years old, earning a podium spot with a silver medal. Looking forward to the next 30 years, she sees herself competing right into her 90s with goals of earning age-group awards and is even considering trying some new sports. Her advice: "Don't dread getting older; embrace it. You can feel so much better and do so much more if you make strength training part of your routine. Start now."

The Baltimore Longitudinal Study on Aging found that aerobic capacity declines through the years (Ferrucci 2008). My client proved this wrong in her case, and her story shows that adding strength training is even more effective than focusing solely on endurance activity. Without cardiorespiratory exercise, the decline in aerobic capacity is accelerated. Why is good aerobic capacity important? It's been shown to reduce the risk of high blood pressure, coronary heart disease, obesity, diabetes, metabolic syndrome, and some forms of cancer (Warburton et al. 2006).

STRENGTH TRAINING IMPROVES POWER DEVELOPMENT

Power is our ability to move a load or our body weight quickly. As already discussed, as people age, one of the top reasons they end up in the hospital is because they fall. Did you know this is due to a lack of power? They can't move fast enough or produce enough power to catch themselves. Improving your power means you'll be able to move quickly to react and catch yourself, along with staying independent as you age. Power development is an important part of your strength training program.

A study published in the *Journal of Strength and Conditioning Research* found that "due to sufficient speed of the lower limb being necessary for functional tasks related to safety (crossing a busy intersection, fall prevention), high-speed power training should be implemented in older adults to improve power" (Fragala et al. 2019).

A client started in her 40s and has been strength training consistently for 22 years. She is a competitive golfer and has been able to stay competitive at 69 years old. One thing she noticed was how over that time she's been able to not only maintain her power when she hits the ball but has also seen improvement. She knows, "If I don't use it, I'll lose it," so she makes sure to use her strength, power, and fitness every day.

STRENGTH TRAINING STRENGTHENS THE PELVIC FLOOR MUSCLES

It is common for women to experience a weakened pelvic floor as they age, whether they've been pregnant, given birth, or not. Difficulty controlling the muscles of the pelvic floor, also known as pelvic floor dysfunction, can lead to urinary incontinence problems, bowel movement difficulty, and lower-back pain. Because the pelvic floor supports the organs in the pelvis, a weak pelvic floor can lead to prolapse, in which the organs start to protrude. Pelvic floor dysfunction can occur due to childbirth or the decrease in estrogen that occurs with perimenopause and menopause, leading to several potential issues: a decrease in the elasticity of the connective tissue, obesity, nerve damage, or injury. You may have heard of or done Kegel exercises, but these are only the beginning of strengthening your pelvic floor.

Throughout this program, follow the cues for the core stability exercises as you learn the plank position, which will translate into all the strength movements. Think of your core as a canister: The deep abdominal muscles make up the front wall, the spinal muscles make up the back, the diaphragm is the top, and the pelvic floor is the bottom. If any of

Common Myths About Women and Strength Training

Myth: Lifting Weights Will Make You Big and Bulky

The goal of this program and the key to aging strong is to build muscle so, yes, you will get stronger, firmer, and fitter. I'm not going to tell you that you won't gain muscle because you will; that's the goal. Hopefully seeing muscle definition on a woman is becoming increasingly common. Strong is the new skinny. I have never in my more than 25-year career seen any woman become big and bulky, looking manly or hulk-like. Getting stronger only makes women more confident in their still very feminine bodies. The only way to look and more importantly feel fit is to build some muscle. You can't be afraid of muscle. In fact, as we age, we need to be afraid of not building muscle because sarcopenia will set in if we don't do something about it. This muscle will give you strong joints that will last for years doing the activities you love in life! You will not look like a man because you lift weights. Get ready to push yourself in the gym, lift enough weight to build muscle, and watch your body change into a fit, strong athlete as you age.

Myth: Women Shouldn't Lift Heavy Weights as They Age

As we age, being weak is infinitely more dangerous than being strong. In these times, women are realizing their strength. We aren't fragile, weak individuals who need help with everything, and as we age, we want to remain as independent as possible. We are perfectly capable and able to lift heavy weights, especially if we've been progressing over time. A characteristic called *training age* refers to how long you've been on a structured, consistent strength training program. Starting now (however old you are) is key to building the strength to take you into your golden years feeling confident in your abilities. Many clients in their 60s and 70s are continuing to hit personal records on their lifts. If you progress properly with the right program—and ideally a coach overseeing your form—you will not get hurt. Build slowly. If you follow the programs in this book, you'll increase your weights each week and each phase with a plus set at the end of each phase to test your strength. Your goal is to challenge yourself to lift heavy with proper form and realize your strength. You have no idea how strong you are, and I can't wait for you to find out!

Myth: Women Get All the Benefits They Need From Aerobic Activities Such as Walking and Running

Cardiovascular activities are good, and living an active lifestyle is great! Walk all the steps, go running if you enjoy it, but realize that none of that is building any strength or muscle. In fact, if you aren't lifting weights and incorporating in progressive overload, which we'll talk more about in chapter 13, you may lose some muscle by running or walking it off. Prioritizing strength training will improve your efficiency with your cardiovascular activities along with all the benefits of lifting weights covered in chapter 2. Sprinkle in some cardio, but make sure it's not your main event. Throughout this book, you'll read client stories who thought cardio, running, or aerobics classes were all they needed until they started strength training and got hooked on that strong feeling.

Myth: Women Don't Need a Specific Program

Yes, we do. We are built differently than men. In general, women have wider hips and breasts that pull our shoulders forward. We are more likely to wear heeled shoes. Many women have babies, but even if you haven't, it's common for women to experience a weak pelvic floor or even prolapse. Some priorities need to be addressed for women that are not as crucial for men, including specific core-strengthening, building the posterior chain to use the glutes and hamstrings better, increasing upper-back strength, and highlighting single-leg exercises since women have a higher likelihood of ACL and hip labrum injuries. The programs in this book will address all these factors.

Myth: Lifting Heavy Weights Will Make You Immobile and Muscle Bound

No, it won't. Immobility happens when you cannot move properly. By performing strength training exercises through a full range of motion, you'll improve your ability to move. By including active stretches as part of your warm-up and recovery with self-massage and flexibility moves, you'll become more mobile as you get stronger! More muscle will not make you less flexible. Not moving will.

Myth: Muscle Turns to Fat if You Stop Strength Training

If you stop strength training, the muscle you've built will provide a buffer so you can take some time off while still getting the benefits of the muscle you have. It will keep you from gaining fat. You will lose muscle over time if you don't use it, but it does not turn into fat.

the sides of the canister are not strong or able to function properly, the pelvic floor will be forced to do more work than it can handle, causing dysfunction. Learning to engage the deep abdominal muscles, strengthen your back muscles, and use your diaphragm will decrease your risk of pelvic floor dysfunction. We'll do all of these in this program. You'll start each workout with diaphragmatic breathing in the warm-up to get you started. If you've been diagnosed with pelvic floor dysfunction, seek out a health care provider's advice in treating it.

STRENGTH TRAINING MAY HELP PREVENT OR DECREASE MENOPAUSE SYMPTOMS

Menopause can come with more than a few symptoms, including hot flashes, weight gain, water retention, insomnia, night sweats, moodiness, and more. Many of these symptoms are caused in a domino effect of hormonal fluctuations. Strength training can help! Strength training can boost testosterone and growth hormone along with helping to decrease body fat. In obese postmenopausal women, adipose tissue is the main source of estrogen biosynthesis, according to a study linking obesity as a risk factor for postmenopausal breast cancer (Cleary and Grossman 2009). Strength training will also increase muscle mass and help optimize hormones to prevent dramatic symptoms of menopause. Of our clients who have been training with us in their 40s through perimenopause and menopause, 95 percent experienced little to no disruptive menopause symptoms. A study published in the journal *Menopause* found that a 16-week exercise program showed a positive effect on menopause-related symptoms among 45- to 60-year-old women (Baena-Garcia et al. 2022).

STRENGTH TRAINING BOOSTS STAMINA AND FUNCTION IN EVERYDAY ACTIVITIES

The byproduct of sarcopenia (muscle loss due to aging) is loss of motor coordination affecting our daily life activities. Many women have rigorous schedules related to their role as the primary caretaker in most households along with their careers, volunteer work, and other community activities. After using the programs in this book, you'll notice a difference in the amount of energy you experience every day.

A client, who is 73 years old, went to her grandkid's volleyball game. On arrival, she noticed there was not a handrail for the higher bleacher seats. Everyone in her age group had camped out on the bottom bleacher, too afraid to try to balance while climbing to a better seat. She, however, was confident in her balance and strength and climbed the bleachers to where she could get one of the best seats in the house to watch her grandkid play.

Being more active in your daily life outside of dedicated workouts, such as walking more or climbing the stairs, will improve your chances of living a longer and healthier life. An article in the *Cleveland Clinic*

Journal of Medicine noted that promoting physical activity in women over 60 helped to decrease their risk of common diseases and injuries as they age (Chavez, Scales, and Kling 2021).

STRENGTH TRAINING REVERSES THE AGING PROCESS

Yes, you *can* turn back the clock! The average woman loses a third of her muscle mass between the ages of 35 and 80. Strength training can reverse this. Every decade after 30 years old muscle mass decreases approximately 3 to 8 percent, and this rate of decline is even higher after age 60, according to a scientific review done on muscle tissue changes with aging (Volpi, Nazemi, and Fujita 2004). Instead of being afraid you'll bulk up, be afraid of losing muscle. Welcome to the only proven way to get younger every day.

STRENGTH TRAINING INCREASES SELF-ESTEEM AND CONFIDENCE

This is by far the most important benefit of consistent strength training. As we age, it's common to lose confidence in our abilities. Strength training increases self-esteem and confidence in women. Almost every client mentioned the word *confidence* when they were interviewed for this book. Strength training was associated with significant improvements in body image, health-related quality of life, and physical activity behaviors, satisfaction, and comfort among a group of 50- to 72-year-old women in a study published in the *Journal of Extension* (Seguin et al. 2013).

Training hard in the gym will make you feel good about yourself, allowing everything else in your life to feel much smoother, including relationships, career, vacations, and other experiences, whatever else you allow it to flow into. The gym isn't just a place you come to work out. The gym is a mindset. It's where you can reinvent yourself. Having a strong, fit body is merely a benefit. A client said, "Showing up for my workout every day is like my job. When I don't work out, I feel out of sorts." I think everyone over 40 needs to treat their workout like their job. It's non-negotiable. This client mentioned her motivation includes "the idea of being able to feel good about my body and confidence that I can do things. Age truly is a number. Friends my same age are unable to do the things I do and that's their choice."

STRENGTH TRAINING AT A GYM PROVIDES SOCIAL INTERACTION

There is a strong positive correlation between social interaction and health and well-being among older adults. Social relationships are consistently associated with biomarkers of health and aging (National Institute on Aging 2021). Positive indicators of social well-being may be associated with lower levels of a chemical called interleukin-6 in otherwise healthy people (National Institute on Aging 2021). Interleukin-6 creates inflammation when there is an injury or infection and is implicated in age-related disorders such as Alzheimer's disease, osteoporosis, rheumatoid arthritis, cardiovascular disease, and some forms of cancer (Omoigui 2007). Having a supportive community where you work out is part of the equation to aging strong. Find a gym that feels like home, as one of our clients called Results Fitness. Another client referred to Results Fitness as her "place to come to connect with other women who are also on the same journey, sharing support and ideas."

CONCLUSION

Most women don't realize they can decrease their risk of osteoporosis, decrease their risk of injuries, increase their metabolism and lose fat, feel younger, function in daily life better, increase their self-esteem, and feel good about themselves by making strength training part of their routine! All these things make aging so much easier and more fun. We can look forward to aging strong instead of dreading it.

CHAPTER 2

THE CARDIO CONUNDRUM

Are you watching what you eat, keeping your calories low, and doing tons of cardio? If so, I bet you're frustrated that you aren't seeing the results you expected from all your efforts. In fact, you may have given up and are now blaming it on being in your 40s, 50s, or whatever stage you happen to be in life. If you grew up doing aerobics classes, "feeling the burn" and addicted to the endorphin-pumping, sweat-inducing loud-music-while-shouting-woo!-feeling, then I'm talking to you. And yes, I was one of those people. I even taught aerobics classes wearing my thong leotard! Ahh, the 80s! Seriously, what was I thinking?

For so long, women thought that the key to looking and feeling the way they wanted was all about burning calories during the workout while eating fewer calories. Spending hours on treadmills and cardio machines watching the calorie counter is what had to be done, right? Wrong. Research shows this simply is not the best way to look and feel fit, healthy, and strong.

One of the landmark studies on interval training pitted 20 weeks of endurance training against 15 weeks of interval training. The number of calories burned by the endurance group equaled a whopping 28,661 calories, while the interval group only burned 13,614 calories (less than half.) Yet the interval training group showed a nine times greater loss of subcutaneous fat than the endurance group, when corrected for energy cost (Tremblay, Simoneau, and Bouchard 1994). Calories burned was not the whole picture.

Actually, every hour of cardio and every calorie you cut over all those years through your 20s and 30s has just finally caught up with you, and now you have to shift how you exercise to build yourself back up. It doesn't get harder as you age; you are just finally paying the price for the years of trying to use a "magic pill" that may have worked temporarily but no longer does. That magic pill could have been the calories burned through the latest trending cardio fad or the fasting craze you got caught up in or some other restrictive diet plan. We'll talk more about nutrition in the next chapter. Whatever it was, if you lost weight, you may have also lost lean muscle tissue, and adding more cardio will not help you get it back. In fact, it could make it worse.

NEAT and Adaptations

NEAT stands for non-exercise activity thermogenesis, and it's also called NEPA, or non-exercise physical activity. These terms describe the calories burned from activities of daily living, not including a purposeful workout session. NEAT is the second largest contributor to your total daily energy expenditure (TDEE) and is made up of the following four areas:

1. Your basal metabolic rate (the calories you burn if you lay on the couch all day, doing nothing), which increases as we add muscle
2. NEAT
3. The thermic effect of food (calories you burn to process the food you eat)
4. Calories burned through exercise

You have to watch your body adjusting for NEAT quite dramatically. This is why extreme diets and too much exercise (particularly excessive cardio) can backfire.

Let's say you burn 2,000 calories per day, and you're eating at a maintenance level. Then you cut 250 calories from your caloric intake and add 250 calories burned from exercise. Now you have a nice 500-calorie deficit and will start losing fat. You're consuming 1,750 and burning 2,250. Then you decide to add another 500 calories of cardio, thinking this will give you a 1,000-calorie deficit and faster results.

The problem is, our metabolism doesn't work like a calculator. Our bodies don't like to change, are extremely smart, and will adjust to maintain homeostasis (keep things the same). In this example, it's very likely your body will adjust the NEAT portion of your TDEE.

After a hard exercise session and burning lots of calories, your body will naturally start to conserve calories. You're a little more tired, so you sit down more. You walk a little slower or park closer. You move a little less. Very quickly, your body is burning maybe 300 to 400 fewer calories per day in this non-exercise activity. Now the 500-calorie deficit you had is almost entirely offset by your body adjusting for NEAT. The body adapts to the extra exercise by downregulating other physiological responses (primarily movement) to keep your deficit at a certain limit.

If you're looking for fat loss, the total caloric burn each day is important, and your total energy expenditure will increase with exercise but tends to plateau at high volumes of exercise as the body adapts to maintain your deficit. So, more is not always better.

This is why we prioritize weight training. It burns calories while you are doing it. Then it keeps burning calories after you've finished and builds muscle, which burns calories at rest, increasing your basal metabolic rate. If you're doing more than four hours of exercise a week, you'll want to keep an eye on your daily non-exercise activity. We've found four hours total to be an ideal amount of exercise to complement an active lifestyle: two or three hours of strength training and one or two hours of high-intensity interval training. Adding more usually leads to an offset with NEAT.

MORE THAN WALKING

Aerobics, walking, spinning, or whatever the hot new cardio workout is often becomes the focus and priority exercise for women in their 40s and beyond because it's what they know. Prioritizing an intense strength training session is rare for women over 40 years old. "I'm too old to do that stuff," one woman shared with me.

At a photo shoot for a women's fitness magazine, a model was filmed while walking to capture someone looking happy, strong, and confident for a cover. Someone on the set said that looks like a photo that could be used for the other magazine that has a target market demographic of women 35 to 54. Sure enough, if you flip through that magazine, you'll mostly see pictures of women walking. This struck me. I realized that if you're 35 or older, the advice in magazines aimed at you is very different than if you are under 35. Once you turn 35, they lead you to believe that walking is enough exercise for you. You're old, after all. Pardon my French, but screw that! Why not step up your workout game as you approach 40 by lifting more, jumping higher, and learning new skills? It's up to you what your 40s, 50s, 60s, and beyond look like.

Living an active lifestyle is encouraged, and as we age, it's easy to become more sedentary. It is a great idea to track your daily activity to be sure you are staying on the move, including walking plenty. If you don't move it, you will lose it. Walking is a good thing. I'm not knocking it. However, if your only form of exercise is a cardiovascular activity without any strength training as you age, you'll find yourself getting weaker, getting injured more often, and having a slower metabolism.

I'm a cardio addict myself. I love running, biking, hiking, and walking. I've completed two Ironman Triathlons that consist of over 2 miles (3 km) of swimming, 120 miles (193 km) of biking, and a full marathon, all in one day. That was 12 to 14 hours of straight cardio in one day, not to mention the hours and hours of training leading up to those events. Every time I ramp up my volume of aerobic activities to the extreme levels that it takes training for an Ironman, I struggle to keep my strength and body composition where I feel best.

In fact, going overboard by doing too much traditional cardio can create hormonal issues, sleep problems, and overtraining symptoms. That is definitely not something you need while you're already navigating perimenopause and menopause.

WHERE CARDIO FITS

So how does cardio fit into an anti-aging workout program? There are obviously benefits to having cardiovascular health, and if you are tight on time, the good news is the strength training programs in this book are

Spotlight on Lauri Struble

Member since 2003

How old were you when you started strength training, and how old are you now?

I was in my 40s when I started, and I just turned 62 years old.

Why did you decide to make strength training a priority?

In college, I became a competitive runner, joining the track and field team and surprising myself that I had a natural talent to run. I placed competitively in my first meet, and I was hooked. During this time, I realized I had an alcohol addiction and decided to get sober. Working out gave me purpose, and being part of a team gave me a reason to get sober. Moving away from self-destructive behaviors, I realized I wanted the freedom to feel confident in my body with myself, no longer wanting to self-medicate. Endorphins became my drug of choice. This year, I celebrate 36 years of being sober.

My workouts for many years consisted of only running, so my body became very thin, and I had no muscle. I realized I needed to start strength training, so I started with crunches, and eventually my first structured strength training program was at Results Fitness.

My mom had severe osteoporosis. I've always been low risk for osteoporosis, and I know it's because I strength train. Where would I be if I wasn't doing that? I'm also on zero medications and want to keep it that way. I continue to strength train because it gives me the freedom to be who I want to be and has a feeling of empowerment. My why is to be a good example for my kids and grandkids.

What was your experience going through perimenopause and menopause?

Menopause symptoms weren't dramatic for me. I had a relatively easy time going through the transition. I experienced some night sweats, but overall, I didn't experience anything debilitating or even worth needing to see a doctor. I attribute that to never missing a workout and taking care of myself.

What results did you get by prioritizing strength training?

Once I started strength training, my fitness levels stayed high, even when I wasn't running. I had more power, my speed increased, I had control going downhill to be able to take advantage of the acceleration, and I started competing. Being strong catapulted me into longer distances. I did my first marathon in my 50s because of consistent strength training twice a week, and I kept doing it right through my marathon training.

When I shifted from running more to make strength training a priority, I found that I'm faster while actually doing less running training. I also noticed my body shape changing with strength training more than anything I've ever done, especially my belly.

I plan to keep running, lifting, and competing. I want to be competing right into my 90s with a goal to keep earning age-group awards and even trying some new sports. I did my first Spartan at 61 years old and earned a spot on the podium for second place.

How many days a week do you lift weights?

I strength train two or three days a week, and three or four days a week, I run two or three miles (3-5 km). I have a routine and make sure to fit it in, no matter what.

What have you found to work for your nutrition?

I have never struggled with nutrition. Eating healthy and fueling my body made sense as I started running and gave up alcohol. I do my best to get enough protein in and eat lots of fruits and vegetables.

What do you recommend to someone who is in their 40s wanting to age strong?

Don't dread getting older; embrace it. You can feel so much better and do so much more than you think. Start now. Realize the benefits of strength training sooner than later and make it non-negotiable.

done to improve your cardiovascular health and help you get stronger. If you don't enjoy cardio, you don't have to do it! Because you'll be doing compound exercises paired with short rest periods, your heart rate will be pumping, and you'll notice that you're out of breath, getting a cardiovascular benefit. These full-body strength training programs two or three days a week as your absolute non-negotiable, number one priority will be the most beneficial to age strong with a healthy body composition and fit cardiovascular health. A study in the *European Journal of Applied Physiology* showed that using a strength circuit of just 12 sets elevated excess post-oxygen consumption (EPOC) for 38 hours after the workout (Schuenke, Mikat, and McBride 2002). Elevating EPOC for 38 hours means your body's metabolism and calories burned stays elevated for almost two days after the workout. You're getting a benefit far beyond the workout itself. This means instead of worrying about the calories burned during the workout, a strength training session will kick your metabolism up for the next day or two!

If you do want to run, bike, hike, or do another aerobic activity because you enjoy it, then, by all means, add it in while keeping strength training as the main focus. Ideally, if you do cardio activities at an intensity that does not tax your system, it can help improve your recovery. Perform cardio below 75 percent of your maximum heart rate so it is part of your active recovery. If you go too hard for too long, you'll end up eating away the hard-earned muscle you are working to build and decreasing your recovery, which will affect your next strength workout.

HIGH-INTENSITY INTERVALS

If you do want to include cardio, performing a high-intensity metabolic interval-style cardio session one or two days a week will be the most effective for boosting metabolism, improving cardiovascular health, and feeling strong. I've included optional metabolic interval workouts for you to include in addition to the strength training workout two or three times a week in chapter 18.

A review study in 2017 compared high-intensity interval training with moderate-intensity continuous training (Wewege et al. 2017). Although both programs improved body composition, the high-intensity interval training required 40 percent less training time. This is a huge factor, especially for busy women wanting the fastest results in the least amount of time. The journal *Menopause* published a study in 2019 showing that postmenopausal obese women doing high-intensity interval training reduced body fat in a third of the time that doing aerobic exercise did (Buckinx and Aubertin-Leheudre, 2019). The study also showed that to build muscle strength, you had to include strength training and couldn't just do high-intensity interval training. Cardio needs to be a side to the priority main event of strength training.

Another important study published in the *Journal of Physiology* in October 2022 showed clear evidence that the only way to preserve muscle tissue as we age is almost exclusively by training our fast-twitch fibers, which means strength training and power development, along with high-intensity interval training (Grosicki, Zepeda, and Sundberg 2022). A quote from the abstract of the study said, "Lifelong aerobic exercise training is unable to prevent most of the decrements in fast fiber contractile function, which have been implicated as a primary mechanism for the age-related loss in whole-muscle power output."

Strength training has to be a part of your anti-aging equation, and if you're going to do one type of cardio for the best results in the least amount of time, high-intensity interval training is your choice. I've included it in the program in chapter 18. The days of doing hours on the cardio machines or trying to keep up with the Broadway dance-caliber aerobics instructor are over!

TRAINING FOR ENDURANCE EVENTS

If you're training for an endurance event or competition, fantastic! I love training for a race and highly recommend having goals on the horizon. As you get stronger, you might find yourself wanting an athletic event to train for, and you should absolutely go for it! I often encourage clients to pick an event and activity that excites and motivates them.

In fact, obstacle course racing is what got me out of my funk as I turned 40. I learned how to climb a rope, swing on monkey bars, and tackle all kinds of new obstacles in my 40s as I started to compete in age-group competitions. This gave my training a new focus that pushed me to get stronger, fitter, and better at running, too. Every year, teams from the gym, mostly women in the 40 to 60 age group, train for a local obstacle course race. They learn new skills and train with a renewed motivation to cross a finish line.

CONCLUSION

Whether you decide to jump into an obstacle course race and learn to overcome the various obstacles or decide to get into golf, pickleball, cycling, or whatever sport you enjoy, pick something that is fun, not that you're hoping to burn calories from. The strength you gain from following the program in this book will make any activity that much more enjoyable. In chapter 1, I covered how strength training will improve your aerobic capacity and efficiency. Strength training will give you the fitness, functional strength, and ability to enjoy whatever activity you'd like to fill your life (time) with.

And no matter what your goal is, always, include strength training at least twice a week to complement the rest of your training and sports. "It's a non-negotiable way of life," as a client put it.

If you find yourself prioritizing walking or another form of steady-state cardiovascular activity, realize that your time can be used much more effectively by performing a full-body strength training program. It may take more effort, but the benefits far outweigh anything else you could spend your time doing.

CHAPTER 3

LIFESTYLE HABITS

The word *diet* has so much negativity associated with it. Most people hear the word and immediately think, "What do I *not* get to eat?" By focusing on what you don't get, you'll immediately want that exact thing!

Let's take a deep breath and realize that we are all on a diet of some sort, because a diet is simply the foods and liquids you eat and drink. For some of us, it's a diet of fruits and vegetables, and for others, it's Pop-Tarts and Cheetos. Be careful about giving your diet more power than it deserves in the form of emotions strongly connected to what you eat. If becoming healthier and stronger is your goal as you age, you'll most likely make a few changes to your current diet.

NUTRITION IS INDIVIDUAL

I asked clients who have been following the strength training program through their 40s, 50s, 60s, and 70s what works for them regarding nutrition. Even though they all had been training with me for years, each had a slightly different answer, although there were commonalities, such as getting enough protein and eating fruits and vegetables. But why didn't they all answer this question the same way? Because every one of us is different. There is no magical nutrition plan. These women have kept it very simple and over time found what works for them. You can too.

Instead of looking at what others are doing, focus introspectively when it comes to your nutrition. How does this food make me feel? Why am I craving that food? What works for me?

In my first book, *The Female Body Breakthrough*, I shared my own experiences with emotions and food. I struggled with a binge eating disorder and eventually bulimia. Both are long behind me now as I enjoy food in a healthy way to fuel my body and connect with friends and family, with everything in moderation. If you're still struggling with food obsession, a binge eating disorder, or any kind of disordered eating heading into your 40s, please seek professional help. Life is too short to let food rule your life.

IMPORTANCE OF GOOD NUTRITION

Many women who gain weight as they approach menopause find that how and where they gain the weight is different than what they experienced when they were younger. Many complain for the first time that they have a belly when they never had that as a problem spot before. A review on understanding weight gain at menopause concluded that the hormonal cascade, which we'll talk more about in chapter 6, is associated with increasing total body fat and abdominal fat (Davis et al. 2012). This chapter is intended to help you do everything in your control to avoid an unwanted increase in body fat by fueling your body to keep your hormones stable, energy levels high, and your body happy.

Many women may have the experience of effectively starving themselves to lose weight, only to regain it and affect their metabolism. In your 20s, 30s, and even sometimes 40s, it's very common to look for a quick fix, a fast 10-pound weight loss or a fat loss blast with the focus on how you look. If you've been comparing yourself to where you were in your 20s or what you did when you were younger, realize that you're in a different body now. Give yourself a clean slate to build toward your next 20 years so that when you're in your 60s, you can look back and realize you've become stronger and healthier every year! It is possible!

I have a client who was featured in my first book. She was in her 40s at that time, having joined Results Fitness three years before the book was published, and is still thriving at 61 years old. (That's her on the cover of this book!) When she joined in her 40s, she had gained 25 pounds (11 kg) and had been trying for 10 years to lose the weight with little success. Initially she started working out with the goal to lose weight. She was disappointed when the weight wasn't coming off as fast as she wanted. She's one of the clients who inspired me to create our Drop Two Sizes program to get women to stop looking at the scale. In fact, I actually took her scale at one point to help her detach from the number on the scale. Instead, she focused on consistently lifting weights two or three times a week, building muscle and losing fat, which really started to shift as she made changes to her nutrition. She tracked her food and increased her protein intake to make sure she was taking in at least a gram of protein per pound of lean body mass.

Over time, her body changed, and she's now fitter and stronger in her 60s than she was when she first started strength training consistently in her 40s. She makes sleep a priority, knowing that it is the key to having energy and a stable mental state. She enjoys a guilt-free nutrition splurge once or twice a week. As she navigated perimenopause and menopause, she had some symptoms like low energy, some hot flashes, and mood swings, but overall, it was mild. Her advice is to make small changes that will gradually build on each other over the years rather than a quick fix and to think about how you want to live in your 50s and 60s. She thinks it's crazy that her friends think she's naturally motivated because she's absolutely not. It's a habit. Train yourself to work out even when you don't have the motivation. You have to work on being motivated. Like a muscle, your motivation will get stronger. You'll struggle with transforming yourself if you depend on always being motivated. It's a choice for every one of us.

Throughout this chapter, I want to give you a lifestyle plan to follow that you can stick to consistently, even when you're not feeling motivated, while enjoying an occasional splurge without guilt. Life's too short to not enjoy the foods you want in moderation.

Fueling your body instead of starving it has never been more important as you enter your 40s, head into perimenopause, and eventually reach menopause. A meta-analysis published in the journal *Menopause* in January of 2023 reviewed 32 different studies and found that nutritional interventions are promising tools for managing mood and anxiety symptoms in women during the menopausal transition and in postmenopausal years (Grigolon et al. 2023). Not eating enough or overdoing processed foods, sugar, and alcohol will wreak havoc on your hormones, which are already on a roller coaster. Feeding processed foods, sugar, and alcohol to a body trying to manage changing hormone levels is a recipe for disaster. Control what you can through your food intake, specifically your blood sugar and the hormones affected by it. Choose foods high in fiber and protein that have anti-inflammatory properties to give yourself a better chance of sailing through your 40s, 50s, and 60s looking and feeling great!

Emotional eating during times of high stress is a common reason for not eating healthy. Stress and anxiety can be high during perimenopause and menopause. Handling this stress and anxiety with junk food and alcohol is a habit. Sound familiar? The good news is that how you manage your stress can be changed. We'll tackle some strategies to make long-term behavior changes beyond just what to eat including learning how to manage stress in healthy and productive ways.

Following a proper nutrition program will ensure you get the most out of your training. If you do not have the right kind of fuel, or not enough fuel, you will not get everything you can out of your training, nor will you have the building blocks to recover from your workouts. When you are putting the physical demands of training on your body and asking it to recover and repair itself, you have to give it what it needs.

LIFESTYLE HABITS TO MASTER

While most of this chapter is about fueling your body properly, other lifestyle choices affect how you feel and what you can do. Many of these lifestyle choices are *habit stacked,* a term from the book *Atomic Habits*

Spotlight on Stephanie English

Member since 2019

How old were you when you started strength training, and how old are you now?

I had worked out off and on, always enjoying being active by playing tennis, running, and walking. The first time I started a serious, structured strength training program, I was 59 years old, and now I'm 63 years old.

Why did you decide to make strength training a priority?

As I was getting older, I started to notice my body changing. The real turning point for me was a full tear of my ACL; I had to stop playing tennis and never fully recovered. I had to find a different way to stay active. I have always been athletic and had a competitive side to me. I would run not because I liked it but to get better at it. The injury left me extremely frustrated that I could no longer do the things to stay active I had done before. Starting a structured strength training program was about finding a different way to keep moving to get strong. Weight loss was definitely a motivation too. I really don't like the way I feel when I'm heavier and wanted to be able to maintain and possibly lose some weight as I got older.

What was your experience going through perimenopause and menopause?

I reached menopause when I was 55 years old and was very lucky to get through it pretty easy with relatively few symptoms. I definitely attribute that to always being active and taking care of myself, always making it a priority to keep my body healthy.

What results did you get by prioritizing strength training?

I noticed I was stronger and able to do things I couldn't do before, even as I entered my 60s. The changes in the appearance of my body really started once I decided to get serious about changing my nutrition. It clicked that I needed to make my nutrition as consistent as my strength training program and truly make this my lifestyle. Overall, joining the gym and learning to lift weights was emotionally remarkable. Being able to move my body, lifting weights, and having the community of incredible people supporting me while seeing the progression is an overall great feeling that I would never give up.

How many days a week do you lift weights?

Two or three days a week.

What have you found to work for your nutrition?

At this point, I eat only unprocessed food in three meals a day with snacks. I always eat breakfast and include protein and vegetables. I used to grab box lunches but realized how much extra stuff was in those, and I no longer wanted to include them as part of my new lifestyle. I have found that tracking helps me a lot. I track my macros, focusing on how many grams of protein (shooting for over 100 grams a day), along with fat and carbs without worrying about calories. I cut out alcohol completely and felt immediately wonderful. I decided to do a hard stop for nine months of no alcohol, realizing that it is actually poison for my body. Now I only enjoy alcohol very occasionally, maybe one or two servings a month if there is a special occasion.

What do you recommend to someone who is in their 40s wanting to age strong?

When you're young, you may not be able to imagine yourself in your 60s, but it's going to be here faster than you think. There is a huge benefit in understanding that as you age, you are always still who you are now. You never feel different, but your body is different. Taxes, death, and our bodies aging are all guaranteed. Having grandkids is a whole other time in your life when you'll want to be active and involved. Make time now to get strong. Find a gym community where you feel safe and show up to do what you need to do. It's not about what the person next to you is doing. Hire a coach you'll build trust with, one who listens and creates your fitness program specifically for you.

by James Clear (2018). For example, if you're not getting enough sleep, you may find yourself craving quick fuel, such as sugar and processed foods. There's no sense in teaching you about nutrition or giving you a list of foods to eat if you're not getting adequate sleep. If you're getting enough sleep, you'll have fewer cravings and are more likely to fuel yourself with healthy, nutritious foods. See how that works? One good habit leads to another!

I want to share my list of top 10 lifestyle habits to master if you want to age strong. These are in order of the habits I'd stack first. We'll then go into more detail later in the chapter.

1. *Sleep.* Dial in your sleep, and everything else in your life will be easier. You'll have more energy. You won't have cravings. You'll recover better and handle stress better.

2. *Less cardio and more progressive weight training.* We covered this in chapters 1 and 2, but it bears repeating. Lift weights! Walking is not enough.

3. *Get hydrated.* Menopausal women commonly don't get the cues to drink enough water. Aim to drink half your body weight in ounces of water every day.

4. *Develop a daily de-stress strategy.* Take the time to slow down. If your body is constantly on the go, your stress hormones will affect you in negative ways, including affecting your other hormones. Find ways to realistically reduce stress.

5. *Prioritize protein.* The recommended daily allowance (RDA) is the bare minimum for what is needed for a sedentary person, and that's not you! You lift weights—heavy weights. An article in the *Journal of Sports Science* concluded that athletes who want to gain muscle and strength need more protein to increase muscle protein synthesis and prevent lean muscle loss, especially when in a caloric deficit (Phillips and Van Loon 2011). The authors suggested aiming for 0.8 to 1 gram of protein per pound of body weight per day. The easiest way to take in this amount of protein is to split it up across your meals. I agree with this amount and in most cases encourage my clients to aim for at least 1 gram per pound of lean body mass per day.

6. *Eat breakfast and a meal every three or four hours.* Keep fuel coming in all day to keep your blood sugar stable. If your blood sugar is stable, your insulin levels are stable. More stable hormones make menopausal symptoms less likely. The weight gain associated with menopause is closely related to your hormones, including insulin, estrogen, and progesterone. Control what you can.

7. *Incorporate fruits, vegetables, legumes, nuts, and grains with as many meals as you can.* All are high in vitamins, minerals, antioxidants, and fiber, which has been closely linked to longevity. As you're going through perimenopause and menopause, you will need more nutrients. Fiber will also help by binding to excess hormones to remove them from the body.

8. *Use supplements.* At our gym, we recommend the core four: protein powder to boost protein intake, especially postworkout; a multivitamin; omega-3 fish oil; and vitamin D. Adding a probiotic to keep your gut happy and a fiber supplement if you aren't getting enough fiber through your diet aren't bad ideas, either.

9. *Think anti-inflammation.* Certain foods create inflammation while others are anti-inflammatory. Include more anti-inflammatory foods in your diet, such as berries, avocados, and fatty fish (salmon, tuna, mackerel, and sardines). I discuss this in more detail later in the chapter.

10. *Prioritize recovery.* Create a strategy that includes some form of daily recovery such as foam rolling, stretching, massage, ice, cryotherapy, an Epsom salt bath, or a vibration platform.

Habit 2 was covered in chapters 1 and 2. Let's look at the other habits in more detail.

Sleep

The body repairs and recovers when it is at rest. Without enough sleep, none of the other healthy habits you engage in will give you the results you could achieve with proper sleep. When you cheat yourself of adequate sleep, you are compromising your immune system, putting yourself at a higher risk of disease, and wreaking havoc on your entire system. One of the most common symptoms of menopause is not sleeping well, usually due to hot flashes or insomnia caused by decreases in estrogen and progesterone. Approximately 75 to 85 percent of menopausal women experience hot flashes, and most have problems sleeping (Schwingl, Hulka, and Harlow 1994).

The hormone melatonin, which is connected to the stress hormone cortisol, is often included in any discussion of sleep problems. If cortisol is high, melatonin will be low. What isn't often talked about is how many other hormones are affected when you aren't sleeping. You'll learn more about the domino effect of hormones in chapter 6; not sleeping can set off a cascade of at least 10 different hormones as well as neurotransmitters. Getting enough sleep can be a game changer to keep your hormones stable and reduce the likelihood of experiencing dramatic menopausal symptoms.

Our bodies are meant to fall asleep when the sun goes down and wake up when the sun rises, which means in the winter we need more sleep than in the summer months (Wiley and Formby 2000). It's also important to get sunlight every day to get your circadian rhythm in sync.

A few things you can do to sleep better include the following:

- Keep your bedroom very cool and dark; 68 degrees is ideal to sleep in. Think of it as your sleep cave.
- Maintain a sleep schedule, going to bed at the same time every night and getting up at the same time every morning, to get your body into a rhythm. If you're not getting eight hours of sleep, gradually go to bed earlier each night.
- Turn off TVs, computers, and phones an hour before bedtime. If you must use one of these devices, wear blue light–blocking glasses.
- Keep the lights in the house at a low level when it's dark outside. Create a calming environment inside your home to signal your body it's closing time.
- Cover clocks, lights, or anything flashing in your bedroom with a small piece of black tape. Any light sensed by your body will inform it that it is not time to sleep.
- Manage your body temperature. Temperature regulation affects your ability to fall asleep easily, especially if hot flashes are hitting. Wear loose clothing made of natural fibers such as cotton

and socks to keep your feet warm. Wearing socks in bed increases blood flow to your feet and heat loss through the skin, which helps lower core body temperature.

- Invest in bedding that feels good and keeps you cool. Look into cooling sheets if you're running hot. For those who experience anxiety, a weighted blanket may help alleviate insomnia. Swedish researchers found weighted blankets improved sleep (Ekholm, Spulber, and Adler 2020). In the study, 120 people received either a light blanket or a weighted chain blanket. After four weeks, those who used the weighted blanket had less insomnia and reduced fatigue, depression, or anxiety during the day.

- Avoid caffeine and alcohol. It doesn't take much alcohol to affect your sleep. A research study published in 2018 showed that women who have as little as one drink before bed can decrease sleep quality by 24 percent; higher amounts decreased sleep quality by 39 percent (Pietilä et al. 2018). Alcohol intake was associated with increasing the sympathetic nervous system, creating a fight-or-flight response, and decreasing the parasympathetic nervous system, which is needed to relax, repair, and recover at bedtime. Alcohol also has to be processed by the liver, which is where hormones are processed. Bogging down your liver with alcohol will guarantee you'll suffer from more menopause symptoms because you're giving your liver more work to do. If you're going to drink alcohol, do it in moderation, not every night, and ideally have your last drink three or four hours before bedtime.

Sleep deprivation has been linked to increasing belly fat by 9 percent over 8 weeks in a study published in the *Journal of American College of Cardiology* (Covassin et al. 2022). A meta-analysis linked lack of sleep to an increased incidence of type 2 diabetes, obesity, and cardiovascular disease (Wiley and Formby 2000). Make quality sleep a top priority!

Hydration

Drinking water is the easiest secret to changing your life, yet it's the hardest to do sometimes. Drinking enough water will keep you energized and assist with appetite control so you won't end up overdoing other foods. According to the Centers for Disease Control and Prevention, 43 percent of American adults don't drink enough water (CDC 2022). Dehydration can affect how your skin looks, how your muscles perform, and your energy levels. Figure out a strategy that works for you to drink your water. Start the day gulping down 20 ounces and then do that again with each meal or get a big water bottle to keep track and sip throughout the day. Adding fruit or flavored salts can help make water easier to drink, too.

De-Stress Daily

The right amount of stress for the right amount of time is good and can strengthen us. Our body creates a spike of cortisol, our stress hormone, when our sympathetic nervous system is kicked into gear with perceived danger in our flight-or-flight state. Then we're supposed to go chill out, letting our parasympathetic nervous system take over, bringing cortisol down while we rest and let our body restore to a state of calm. Each stressor will make us stronger if we have both of these. Unfortunately, most people are in a fight-or-flight state from the moment their alarm goes off, and it escalates throughout the day without any parasympathetic time. Then they lie in bed at night, wondering why they can't sleep.

Exercise is also a form of stress. If you add it on top of an already stressed-out body, you won't get the results you're looking for. In fact, chronic high cortisol can cause anxiety, depression, headaches, nerve problems, digestive issues, a weakened immune system, heart disease, high blood pressure, high blood sugar, and—you guessed it—more menopause symptoms (Cleveland Clinic 2021). Make it a habit every day to decompress in some way. A gratitude journal, meditating, deep breathing, playing with your pet, or prayer are all good choices.

Eat Enough Protein

Reasons to eat an adequate amount of protein include getting amino acids to help build and repair muscle, to slow down the blood sugar spike when eaten with carbohydrates, to fill you up with only 4 calories a gram, and to burn more calories because protein has a higher thermic effect.

Building muscle is crucial to an anti-aging regimen. If you don't actively try to maintain or build lean muscle mass, then you could find yourself losing muscle and strength as you age, a condition also known as sarcopenia. Eating enough protein has been shown to help build muscle and strength and is necessary, according to an article published in *Nutrients* in 2018 (Stokes et al. 2018).

Plus, if you are trying to lose body fat, high protein intake can help prevent muscle loss while you are in a caloric deficit. A study looking at increased protein intake during weight loss found that participants who took in 1 gram of protein per pound of body weight (or approximately 35% of calories from protein) maintained lean body mass while in a caloric deficit significantly better than those who took in only 0.45 grams of protein per pound of body weight (or 15% of total calories from protein per RDA standards) (Mettler, Mitchell, and Tipton 2010). If you're cutting calories, bump up that protein to age strong! I recommend a minimum of 1 gram of protein per pound of lean body mass per day.

Eating protein while trying to lose body fat also works to keep you feeling full, reduce your appetite, and boost calories burned through its higher thermic effect of food, according to a study published in 2004 that looked at the effects of high-protein diets on thermogenesis, satiety, and weight loss (Halton and Hu 2004).

Overall, a higher-protein diet will equal enhanced weight loss, stable blood sugar, and better recovery. In a 2021 review on nutrition in menopausal women, the authors discussed the need for increased protein as we age because skeletal muscle reduces its capacity to activate protein synthesis, and a higher protein intake is associated with being less frail, having higher lean body mass, and 32 percent better physical daily function in postmenopausal women (Silva et al. 2021). Aim for 4 to 6 ounces of protein at each meal, which is the size and thickness of your palm and equals about 25 to 35 grams of protein. Throughout this book, you'll hear stories from our clients who track their protein intake, with some aiming to take in 100 grams or more per day.

Eat Breakfast and Then Eat Every 3 or 4 Hours

Fasting has become all the rage, yet over time, I have not seen better results with our clients who fast. In fact, I think it could create more problems, especially for women entering into perimenopause and menopause, because it can have a negative effect on hormones and metabolism. A 2018 study observed 11 overweight women doing a two-day fast and found that they had an increase in sympathetic nervous activity or stress (Solianik and Sujeta 2018). Stress causes an increase in cortisol, which can create a cascade of other hormone fluctuations. This response has not been found in men, suggesting that fasting triggers this stress response in women while men don't experience it. According to an analysis published in the *Annual Review of Nutrition* in 2021, intermittent fasting is not better than regular dieting (Varady et al. 2021). Both resulted in the same amount of weight loss, changes in blood pressure, cholesterol, and inflammation. It's simply a different way of getting the same result, not a superior way. Fasting is a way to cut your overall calories, which can be done while still eating throughout the day.

The problem with fasting is that I have seen it set women up for a binge, creating a starve-and-binge cycle that can be extremely problematic in combination with the hormonal fluctuations that accompany perimenopause and menopause. There are exceptions to this because everyone is different, and I'm encouraging you to find what works for you. Some clients have found that eating dinner early, or not eating before a morning workout for those who aren't breakfast people, works for them without triggering a binge or stress response. Overall, I've seen the best results with most clients when they make it a habit to eat breakfast in the morning and then keep their blood sugar and therefore insulin stable throughout the day, fueling themselves with protein, vegetables, fruits, and healthy fats. Consider the following:

- A study published in 2021 found that postmenopausal women who eat more often, including snacking more and increasing daily fiber intake, can have a lower body mass index (Skoczek-Rubińska et al. 2021).

- A previous study showed a group eating six meals per day lost more fat than a group eating two meals per day, despite calories being equal (Iwao, Mori, and Sato 1996).

- Another study showed irregular meal intake created a lower thermic effect of feeding than a regular meal pattern of six meals per day despite total meals per week being the same (Farschchi, Taylor, and Macdonald 2004).

- A study showed adults who ate four meals a day and switched to three meals a day gained body fat and weight despite calories being the same (Louis-Sylvestre et al. 2003).

Skipping meals may increase your likelihood of metabolic syndrome and make the belly fat issue that so many menopausal women struggle with even worse.

Eat More Plant-Based Foods

Incorporate fruits, vegetables, legumes, nuts, and grains into as many meals as you can to get plenty of fiber each day. Eating according to a Keto diet or the low-carb craze has become very popular; however, this way of eating may result in a diet without enough fiber. On the other hand, plant-based diets are also very popular and a great way to think of how to eat. Considering these two extreme ways of thinking may give us a path down the middle.

Here's the thing: Plant-based doesn't mean no meat. Plant-based means that most of your plate includes fruits, vegetables, and whole grains. Fruits and vegetables many phytonutrients, fiber, vitamins, and minerals, including antioxidants that will reduce the risk of disease. These are crucial to keep your body functioning optimally and to set you up to age strong for years to come. Vitamin D, magnesium, zinc, and vitamin C all help create new cells to repair and rebuild your muscle tissue and bone mass. Making a plate of food that has a base of fruits and vegetables along with high-quality protein and anti-inflammatory fats is exactly what your body needs to age strong. Don't be afraid of carbohydrates in the form of whole grains, fruits, and vegetables that provide fiber, vitamins, and nutrients.

Eating enough daily fiber has been closely connected to improving longevity and even decreasing symptoms of menopause (Skoczek-Rubińska et al. 2021). Fiber helps your body absorb all the nutrients it needs and helps bind up extra estrogen as your body is breaking it down to leave the body while bulking up your stools. A study published in the journal *Menopause* showed that consuming more dietary fiber reduced hot flashes by nearly 20 percent (Grigolon et al. 2023). Fiber helps to keep your gut microbiome healthy so your good bacteria will flourish to be able to digest and get the most out of your food. Shoot for a minimum of 25 grams of fiber a day.

Supplementation

Another important part of a healthy exercise and nutrition plan is supplementation. Did you know that most people do not have sufficient levels of vitamins and minerals for optimal health? Many people are deficient in vitamin D, which is crucial to having an optimal immune system (Lerchbaum 2014). If you end up getting sick or injured and have to try to play catch-up to get the nutrients in, you'll take longer to fight it off or to repair your body after trauma. It's better to always be ready instead of having to get ready once you're sick. Supplements allow you to fill the gaps you might be missing with your nutrition. These are not magic pills; they are meant to supplement a healthy nutrition and exercise plan. Supplements are an important part of a healthy plan, but don't expect them to do the work for you. Eating a nutritious diet full of fruits, vegetables, high-quality protein, and fats is important while taking a high-quality multivitamin to act as an insurance policy, filling any gaps that you might be missing.

What should be in your supplement arsenal as you head into your 40s, 50s, and 60s? A vitamin D supplement and high-quality omega-3 fish oil are the superpower supplements I recommend. More on each of these in the next sections.

Multivitamins

A daily multivitamin is an insurance policy to cover your bases in case you missed anything in your food. It's crucial that you get extra vitamins, minerals, and nutrients to repair and rebuild cells as you are aging. Giving your body everything it needs will ensure you can keep growing muscle, get strong, and build bone mass. One research study with 216 women showed taking a multivitamin improved cognitive performance, fatigue, and mood, which are all possible symptoms of perimenopause and menopause (Haskell et al. 2010). Your multivitamin should include zinc, magnesium, and vitamin C. When it comes to supplement companies, there are very few brands I'll take and recommend to our clients. Metagenics, a pharmaceutical-grade supplement, is the brand we use ourselves and offer in our facility. Be careful about getting your supplements for low prices at places like the grocery store. You'll want to make sure that the supplements you are purchasing have third-party testing to ensure that what's on the label is what's in the bottle.

EPA and DHA Omega-3 Fish Oil

Our cell walls are made up of fatty acids that need to constantly be replaced. If we are not taking in enough good fats, our bodies will not be able to keep our cells from becoming rigid and more prone to disease. In addition, omega-3 fats are anti-inflammatory, helping with everything from depression to decreasing heart disease (Chae and Park 2021). The anti-inflammatory effects will help with symptoms of estrogen dropping. Estrogen is an anti-inflammatory hormone so as it drops entering into menopause, you may experience symptoms of inflammation such as joint pain. Taking omega-3 fish oils will help combat that. Research studies have shown women in menopause and postmenopause who take omega-3 fish oil supplements have less depression and fewer night sweats (Mohammady et al. 2018).

Vitamin D

Vitamin D has become a supernutrient as more research proves it to be the answer to keeping us healthy, improving mental health, helping absorb calcium and phosphorous critical for building bone, boosting the immune system to decrease your risk of respiratory infections, and even reducing cancer cell growth and inflammation (Lerchbaum 2014). Besides vitamin D's well-known and researched role in calcium metabolism and building bone, low vitamin D levels have been associated with a higher risk of cardiovascular disease, metabolic syndrome, type 2 diabetes, cancer, depression, impaired cognitive function, and increased mortality (Caron-Jobin et al. 2011). Take your vitamin D! Furthermore, two studies showed that taking a vitamin D supplement will help decrease abdominal fat, which could be beneficial since having a belly is one of the most common complaints of women as they age (Seo et al. 2012; Rosenblum et al. 2012). It's a good idea to discuss vitamin D supplementation with your doctor, who can test your levels to find out if you are deficient and may need more than the minimum dose to give you a specific recommendation. At a minimum, supplement with 600 IUs of vitamin D a day.

Consume Anti-Inflammatory Foods

It's true our bodies don't tolerate what they used to, and we need to take advantage of foods that will make us feel better, not worse. Inflammation is one of the key reasons for several diseases as we age. Anything ending in "-itis" is inflammation, including one of the most common diseases almost everyone over 40 will experience: arthritis. By consuming foods that have anti-inflammatory properties every day, your cells can stay fluid instead of becoming rigid as you age. Increasing scientific evidence has shown that compounds such as flavonoids—found in fruits, vegetables, and legumes—can have anti-inflammatory properties, along with arachidonic acid, EPA, and DHA found in fatty fish (Calder 2010; Maleki, Crespo, and Cabanillas 2019).

Here are some of the top anti-inflammatory foods to include in your diet:

- Fatty fish such as salmon, tuna, mackerel, and sardines
- Berries
- Avocados
- Green leafy vegetables such as spinach, kale, and broccoli
- Olive oil
- Nuts such as almonds and walnuts

These are foods that can cause inflammation:

- Processed carbohydrates, especially those that contain sugar or high-fructose corn syrup, such as breads and pastries
- Fried foods
- Alcohol
- Soda
- Processed meat such as hot dogs and sausage
- Margarine or other trans fats

Let's talk more about alcohol consumption. I already discussed its effects on sleep, but there's more. Many of my clients who enjoyed an adult beverage regularly noticed that drinking alcohol was not working for them as they entered perimenopause and menopause. If they were used to enjoying a nightly glass of wine or two or a night out on the weekend, they found that their hormonal fluctuations and symptoms were exacerbated by alcohol intake. This is due to the following:

- Even before perimenopause, women are not as tolerant of alcohol as men. Women have less of the enzyme that breaks down alcohol and typically a smaller body composition. Men tend to have more muscle, which helps them metabolize alcohol easier (another reason to hit the weights if you enjoy adult beverages sometimes).

- As we age, the water volume in our body drops so we are unable to dilute alcohol as well. If you're going to drink alcohol, be sure to stay hydrated by alternating with a glass of water.

- Hormones such as estrogen and progesterone are processed in the liver, and these hormones break down more as your levels drop during menopause. Since your body treats alcohol as a poison, your liver has to divert its attention from its other priorities to process it. If you're drinking more than one serving of alcohol per day, you are keeping your liver from processing the estrogen and progesterone that needs to be a priority.

- A study suggested alcohol use had a positive correlation with increased hot flashes (Schwingl, Hulka, and Harlow 1994).

- Alcohol consumption will raise your blood sugar, which raises your insulin levels and sends your body into a cascade of hormonal fluctuations.

- You won't sleep as well at night. It's been shown in the research that having alcohol before bed affects your sleep (Pietilä et al. 2018).

Everyone's body metabolizes alcohol differently, so stay in tune with how you feel the next day and whether you experience worse menopausal symptoms or not. For women, moderate alcohol consumption is considered seven servings or less a week with the idea being no more than one or two servings a day. If enjoying an adult beverage is on your list of non-negotiables, keep your alcohol servings to no more than one or two a day, hydrate alongside your beverage, have your last drink before 8:00 p.m. so the alcohol is less likely to affect your sleep, and always eat protein first to slow down the blood sugar spike.

A client joined the gym when she was 45 years old, and she is now 58 years old. She experienced one year of really tough menopause symptoms, including extreme moodiness. To manage her symptoms, her doctor recommended she come to the gym more often because it was the one thing that made her symptoms better. What a great doctor! Lifting weights was helping her de-stress while also giving her an endorphin kick and helping to stabilize the hormonal fluctuations causing her mood swings. She stepped up her strength training from twice a week to three times a week. Even her family would ask, "Did you go to the gym today?" if they noticed she was extra moody, and the answer was usually not yet.

She also noticed that her habit of enjoying a glass or two of wine a couple nights a week before bed was always followed by the days that she had the worst mood swings. As she started to connect this, she decided to give up alcohol all together. She slept better without alcohol and felt her moods were more stable. She was able to navigate menopause without hormone replacement therapy, even though her blood tests showed her estradiol crashed from 771 to 75 from the start of menopause to it being over. This explained the mood swings she had experienced. Now at 58 she continues to lift weights, competes in obstacle course races, and no longer indulges in adult beverages knowing she doesn't feel her best when she does.

Her story is not uncommon. In fact, another client was finding the same thing as she realized her habit of nightly wine, especially during the pandemic, was not healthy. Many people found themselves turning to alcohol in 2020 more than usual. She decided to eliminate it for nine months to get out of the habit and instantly felt "wonderful." She now only enjoys a glass or two at special occasions, knowing that it is not going to help her feel her best. Some of the behaviors and habits that worked for you before may no longer work for you now. By making the commitment to listen to your body and find what works, you could end up healthier, stronger, and feeling better than you ever have as you transition through menopause.

Recovery Strategies

You can't train hard and expect to improve if you're not giving your body the time and resources it needs to create that adaptation. The harder and longer the training session, the deeper and longer that recovery curve. Make recovery as much a priority as training. I already covered getting enough sleep every night, hydrating, and consuming enough protein, which are all important keys to full recovery. In addition to a good night's sleep, your recovery program should include one of the following each day:

- Foam rolling or other self-myofascial release
- Massage
- Dedicated flexibility and mobility session
- Epsom salt bath
- Compression recovery
- Ice
- Cryotherapy or cold immersion
- Low-intensity activity to get the blood flowing

If you are going to follow the Age Strong training program, also follow this Age Strong recovery program to maximize your results.

CONCLUSION

After reading through this chapter, go back and pick one or two of the topics to focus on making some changes. If you aren't getting enough sleep, start there. If you aren't eating enough protein or drinking enough water, start tracking your intake or simply fill up your water bottle and start gulping it down! The action steps in this chapter will help your overall health and fitness and recovery from your workouts and therefore enhance your results from this program.

PART II

PREPARE FOR POSITIVE CHANGE

CHAPTER 4

SET POWERFUL GOALS

Why do we stop doing the things that make us feel good? Over the years, we learn that eating healthy foods, drinking water, and avoiding junk food makes us feel good, yet these are some of the very habits we still have to work to change. Why?

In *Switch: How to Change Things When Change is Hard* (2010), authors Chip and Dan Heath give two reasons why it's difficult to change:

1. Humans are emotional creatures. As a rule, high emotions make it difficult to think logically.

2. Our environments or situations make change difficult.

The only way to succeed long term is to remove the temptations and put strategies in place when we're thinking logically to outsmart our emotional side and make it easier to stay on the path to feeling our best.

In *The Happiness Hypothesis: Finding Modern Truth in Ancient Wisdom*, Jonathan Haidt (2006) shares the three steps for habit change:

1. Obtain clear directions. This reduces mental paralysis. You will find clear directions in this book.

2. Find an emotional connection to the goals you set, the more meaningful the better. This is what we'll attempt to do in this chapter.

3. Reduce the obstacles, tweak the environment, and make the journey as easy as possible. The more you have to grit and grind your way through, the less likely you'll be to stick with it long term. Tips for reducing obstacles, changing the environment, and making the journey easy were included in the previous chapter.

Age can be a slippery slope as we become more sedentary, experience more stress, and develop or continue poor sleep habits while increasing the consumption of processed foods, alcohol, and sweets, perhaps making us feel fatter, weaker, or slower; experience more pain; and feel tired. It's common to chalk it up to this being what getting old feels like. It doesn't have to be that way.

Mindset is one of the most important factors to consider as you go through perimenopause and menopause. Your body is listening to everything you are saying in your mind and taking it as a command. If you think getting older is going to be hard, it probably will be. If you decide to set goals to get fitter, stronger, and healthier and get even more out of experiencing life as you age, guess what? You will!

SET SPECIFIC GOALS

Are you ready to change? What can you expect? What will motivate you to make these changes long term?

Setting goals and getting focused might be the most important step in this process, even though it has nothing to do with exercise or nutrition. This simple yet critical step must be completed before you lift a weight or start a nutrition program. If you successfully complete this step, the training will come easy. If you ignore this step, you will have a much harder time following through on new lifestyle changes long term.

Most people won't take the time to actually set goals. By thinking through what your future looks like if you stay on the path you are on versus making changes to finally look and feel the way you want to, you'll find making those changes will be much easier.

A client stated, "It's not hard." I interrupted and said, "You mean that you have to choose your hard, right? You either choose the hard path of getting out of shape, losing strength and muscle every year, and becoming more prone to injury and ultimately hospitalization OR you choose the hard work of making changes starting a strength training program and pushing yourself to get fitter, stronger, and healthier now." She replied, "No, it's not hard. People need to realize working out consistently and eating well most of the time really isn't hard." To her, it's not hard because at this point, she's connected how good she feels as she's getting older to the effort she puts in. In comparison, the amount of work she is doing doesn't feel hard compared to how great she feels. To her, "It's not hard" to lift weights two or three days a week and fuel her body with foods that make her feel good. The more you can connect what you'll gain by making changes, identifying your powerful why and how good you'll feel, you will also come to think, "This really isn't hard. Why don't more people do this?"

By getting clear on what you want from living a healthy, fit lifestyle and identifying the driving force behind your training, you'll have tapped into unstoppable motivation. Take your time and do all the exercises in this chapter. You will set yourself up for success by getting your mind in the right place heading into this journey.

Realizing you are able to make changes to reach specific goals has been shown in research to actually slow the inflammatory burden in older adults, according to a study published in the *Journal of Applied Gerontology* (Hladek et al. 2022). By focusing on improving yourself and seeing yourself make progress physiologically, you'll become healthier physically and mentally!

The idea of setting a goal to be able to do something, experience something, or feel something is so much more compelling than a number on a scale or a certain size of clothing. I love the quote by Lexie and Lindsay Kite (2020): "Your body is an instrument, not an ornament."

WHAT IT MEANS TO BE IN SHAPE

At the beginning of the book, I shared my story of turning 40 and my surprise when I realized I was on the same slippery slope many of my clients were on. I set the goal to start racing in obstacle course races as an age-group competitive athlete, wanting to stand on my first podium. This goal to be able to master the obstacles and keep up with the other competitors motivated me to push myself to make changes. Having identified races and knowing I'd be standing at the start line alongside other fierce 40- through 49-year-old women gave me the external accountability I needed to climb off the downhill slide! My workouts took on a new motivation and focus, I made better choices with my nutrition, and suddenly recovery was a really big priority in my schedule. Standing on my first podium after putting in the work felt really good!

A few years later in 2020 when the pandemic hit, I decided to switch gears and train for my second Ironman Triathlon. It had been 14 years since my first one. The decision to train for an Ironman was more for my head than anything; it gave me a reason to go on very long bike rides to handle the stress of my business being closed. My training shifted gears, mostly including long-endurance swimming, biking, and running, plus strength training three days a week.

As I was finishing my training and getting ready to race, someone said to me, "That's so amazing! You're in the best shape of your life! What will you do next?" The question made me ask myself, "Am I in the best shape of my life?" I could complete an Ironman Triathlon; I was in shape to do that. But when I went to the obstacle course World Championships, I was in a different "best shape of my life." Completing an Ironman requires a focus on endurance; completing an obstacle course requires a focus on strength and skill. Being in the best shape of our lives is a definitive destination, and I'm not sure we ever really reach it. It's a flexible concept that can change depending on what we want to do.

Often a client will join Results Fitness with the goal to get in "the best shape of their life." What an incredible goal to have! I really hadn't thought about being in the best shape of my life while I was focused on being able to swim 2.2 miles (3.5 km), cycle 112 miles (180 km), and run a marathon with the bigger goal of getting through the pandemic mentally and physically better off than I started it.

Spotlight on Mel Johnson

Member since 2000

How old were you when you started strength training, and how old are you now?

I was 46 years old when I started, and I turn 70 years old this year. I was one of the first clients at Results Fitness when they opened and am so glad I started there when I did.

Why did you decide to make strength training a priority?

I'm an endurance athlete, a competitive golfer, and I enjoy being active in life. I used to only run for exercise. I realized I needed to start doing something else as I got older to get stronger and work my body in different ways. I found that doing only repetitive running didn't work for me as I aged, so I needed to switch it up. I really wanted to stay fit and flexible. I don't stretch on my own. I think that flexibility was the aspect I most needed in golf and life. A strength training routine combined with stretching is the perfect combination.

What was your experience going through perimenopause and menopause?

Mine was not a typical menopause experience since I had a hysterectomy at 38. I was on HRT from that point on, so I never really had dramatic symptoms. I went off HRT in my early 50s and switched to taking bioidentical hormones, which I've been taking ever since and feel good on. I have a doctor I really trust and check in with my primary care physician regularly.

What results did you get by prioritizing strength training?

I have confidence in my daily living and am able to do the things I want to do without second-guessing myself. I look at my mom, who is 96 years old, and think had she gone to the gym, life would be very different for her. She's very weak and always has been. I don't ever want to feel weak, so I love that I'm gaining strength as I get older. I surprise people that I can do 30 push-ups. My friends are amazed at what I can do. They could too if they decided to. At the golf course, I'm often used as the example of how to swing. Strength training helps me to stay balanced since I'm always swinging in one direction. I have gained power in my golf distance along with flexibility in my hips, legs, and back. I don't know if I could play golf without the workouts I do at Results Fitness, because it has kept me more agile as I age. At 70 years old, I'm still golfing, hiking, and living an active lifestyle while being able to play an active role in my grandkids' lives.

How many days a week do you lift weights?

Twice a week.

What have you found to work for your nutrition?

I'm really careful to eat very healthy because as I got older, I did notice belly fat becoming an issue that I never had before. I eat a lot of protein and a lot of veggies, always trying to make the healthiest choice possible. I always eat breakfast, usually a protein bar on the go, and get at least three healthy meals a day.

What do you recommend to someone who is in their 40s wanting to age strong?

Your life is your oyster. You have to decide what you want to get done. Nobody's going to do it for you. At any age, you can start something new. Find a gym like Results Fitness where you can get good guidance to help you to accomplish what you want in life.

The question is, in the best shape of your life for what?

The human body has always fascinated me because it is an incredible machine that we can train to do anything. I truly believe anything is possible, no matter your age or athletic history. I've had the opportunity to follow specific training programs for many different goals, and throughout every one of them I've learned new things about myself and my body.

When I shifted from focusing on losing weight or getting a six-pack to what my body can do, using my body as an instrument to conquer obstacles, feeling empowered, lifting twice my body weight, or crossing the finish line of a race, I experienced my body getting stronger, fitter, and leaner, including seeing visible muscle and getting a six-pack while preparing for a specific goal. Focus on what your body is capable of, not what it looks like.

Although I was ready to complete an Ironman Triathlon, I was *not* the strongest I'd ever been. That would be when I trained for a powerlifting meet. Or when I went to the Spartan World Championship and was able to tackle any obstacle with confidence with my best strength-to-weight ratio to date. Neither of those times could I have completed an Ironman Triathlon.

I'm also not the leanest I've ever been, because that would be when I trained for a figure competition and really dialed in my training and nutrition with the goal of reaching a specific body composition and "look." But I know I couldn't have run a half marathon, let alone an Ironman at my leanest, most depleted and unhealthy. But I looked good in a bathing suit on stage.

Chasing the goal of being lean or weighing a certain number doesn't lead to being able to **do more** with your incredible machine of a body and instead can lead to a distorted body image, especially when maintaining that state is unrealistic. Focusing on what your body is capable of rather than how it looks will lead to realizing your body's potential to do things you never thought you could do and have the experiences of a lifetime, along with better health and happiness, while your body transforms to become the athlete you need to become for your specific goal. Being able to "do" life is so much more important as you age than a number on the scale or how you look.

Training for an Ironman is another extreme, requiring a very high volume of steady-state cardio beyond what's needed for health. You consume more carbohydrates, which is not ideal for improving body composition because you end up trying to maintain muscle while your body becomes efficient at storing energy for the really long workouts you're doing. A lot of people think, "I'll train for an Ironman or a marathon to reach the best shape of my life," but that isn't necessary unless you want to be able to cross the finish line of an Ironman or marathon to get that feeling of accomplishment on the journey of the training you have to put in.

STRENGTH ABOVE ALL ELSE

Every goal I've trained for has had strength training as a priority. Even while training for an Ironman, I still did strength training three times a week to do everything I could to maintain my muscle and keep my joints strong to handle the impact of 140.6 miles (226 km) while also being able to generate as much power as I could to propel myself forward as I swam, biked, and ran.

Strength training truly is the cheat code. If you've set the goal to be in the best shape of your life, let's get more specific and decide what do you want to be in the best shape of your life for. What's important to you right now?

Focusing on what your body can do rather than how you look will set you up for a healthier relationship with your body. Are you able to do the things you want to do to enjoy life and live an active lifestyle? Be able to hike with your family? Water ski again? Is it to be able to complete an Ironman Triathlon or win a powerlifting meet? Training for an event or experience is much more powerful motivation than looking a certain way. Is it to be superhuman with a robust immune system able to fight off sickness and disease and with a body composition that is optimal for health and reduced inflammation? Believe me, you don't need to train for an Ironman to achieve the best shape of your life.

Strength is usually the limiting factor for many people for any goal. Once you decide what you want to do, start by building the strength you'll need first to give you the functional ability to do whatever it is you want to do while moving efficiently, without hurting yourself.

Step one is to build base strength. Follow the base phase of the program in this book and then work up to some of the benchmarks set by the end of the 16-week program: hold a plank for a minute, perform 10 bodyweight push-ups, squat half your body weight, deadlift 1.5 times your body weight, perform a bodyweight chin-up, etc. I like to think of getting clients to a point where they are six weeks out from anything (although if an Ironman is on your goal list, we'll need more than six weeks).

The two types of goals are outcome goals and process goals, and you'll want to have both. Outcome goals describe the result or destination you want to achieve, such as the benchmarks listed in the previous

Set an Outcome Goal

First, find yourself an inspiring journal to use for the 16 weeks you're following this program. This will be separate from your workout tracking. You will use this journal to keep track of your habits. In the journal, answer this question: What do you want to do with your incredible body? This question purposely does not ask what you want to look like or how much weight you want to lose. This question is purely to get you thinking about the way you want to feel doing the things you want to be able to do and experience. This is your outcome goal. Get specific because this is your powerful goal. The clearer it is, the easier it will be for you to stay focused on it.

What do you want to do with your incredible body?

Next answer this question: Why do you want to reach this goal? Dig deep and really think about why. If you don't have an important enough why that allows you to tap into your intrinsic motivation, it will be very hard to stay on the path to get to where you want to go.

Why do you want to reach this goal?

There are two types of motivation: intrinsic and extrinsic. Intrinsic comes from inside; you do something because it's important to you to feel a certain way. Extrinsic motivation is based on an external reward or gain, a dangling carrot for you to chase. It's not a bad idea to have both, but research confirms that intrinsic motivation leads to the most positive long-term outcomes. A review published in 2012 that included 66 studies showed consistent positive results for intrinsic motivation and exercise (Teixeira et al. 2012). This question will help you get in touch with your intrinsic motivation.

On a scale of 1 to 10, how important is your why? On a scale of 1 to 10 how motivated are you?

If you don't score 10 out of 10 for both these questions, consider whether your outcome goal is important enough for you to make some major changes. If it's not important enough and you're not motivated, that's OK. Rethink why you picked up this book and what really matters to you. That is what you have to do to be able to age strong.

Don't wait until Monday or next week or next month. Start now. What action can you take right now to move toward your powerful outcome goal?

paragraph. We don't have as much control over outcome goals day to day, but they can be used to set the destination. Process goals describe daily actions undertaken to reach your outcome goal. You have total control over whether you do these or not. If you do follow through and complete your process goals, you are more likely to accomplish your outcome goal.

OUTCOME GOALS

Let's get specific and set some goals! Setting an outcome goal is putting the destination in place so you can set the path to make it a reality. The path will include process goals or action steps. In chapter 3, we covered the lifestyle habits that will lead you down the path to aging strong. The outcome goal takes you one step further to connect emotions to why you want to age strong. This exercise is what will set you up for success on this program. By setting the destination, you make it clear where you want to go and why.

ASSESS WHERE YOU ARE

The next step is to take inventory of where you are now. Think through some of your current frustrations, pain, health issues, and weaknesses that you want to move away from. These might include being overweight, feeling tired, being moody, having no energy, feeling out of breath when you walk up stairs, and so on. What are the benefits of continuing the path you're on? What are the costs? Write your answers in your journal.

By digging into what makes you unhappy now and the costs of staying there, you'll be motivated to move away from those issues by taking action each day down the path to reach your goals. Remember that your habits up until this point equal the result of where you are right now. It's a simple equation.

$$X + Y + Z = \text{result}$$

no sleep + processed food + no exercise = tired, weak, grumpy, craving more junk food

8 hours of sleep + whole foods w/ plenty of protein + working out two or three times a week = energized, strong, happy, and confident

Once you know your starting point and your destination, you can figure out how to change the coordinates or equation (habits) from what you've been doing that landed you where you currently are to new coordinates (habits) that will lead you to your new goals.

Pilots are taught the rule of 1 in 60; what seems like a small error—veering 1 degree off course—will cause you to land at a destination 1 mile (2 km) off for every 60 miles (97 km) flown. After a mile, 1 degree starts to make a pretty big difference, and you're off by more than 90 feet (27 m)! This means you'll miss the runway and could end up landing on a lake or crashing into a mountain. If you are 1 degree off course while flying around the equator, you'll land almost 500 miles (805 km) off target! Completely off target from your destination!

> ## Big doors swing on small hinges.
> Clement Stone

The point is that small actions accumulated over a very long time make a huge difference. By knowing where you are and where you want to go, you can avoid veering off course over time and stay on the path to get to your destination.

PROCESS GOALS

Process goals give you specific actions to check off daily, weekly, or monthly to make your outcome goal a reality. You can control these process goals or action steps each day to make your outcome become more likely to happen. Review the lifestyle habits discussed in chapter 3 and identify those that will have the biggest impact in helping you get to your destination.

Set Process Goals

Let's write down some specific process goals. Answer these questions in your journal:

What are some of the changes you want to put into place?

What are the benefits of making these changes?

What are the costs?

Next to each change you want to make, assign a number from 1 to 5 based on how important that habit is to you, 1 being not so important and 5 being very important. Then assign another number, 1 to 5, based on how confident you are that you can do it, 1 being not confident and 5 being very confident. Add these two numbers to get a number out of 10 for each change. The habits that scored the highest will be your focus first to get your momentum heading toward your goal.

CONCLUSION

If you read through this chapter and thought you'd do its tasks later, stop right now and block out a time on your schedule to sit somewhere quiet and really think through your answers and most importantly your why. Early morning, when nobody else is up, is my favorite time for this kind of deep introspective work. Early morning is also when your logical, conscious mind is still not fully awake to tell you nonsense like, "You'll never be an athlete. What are you thinking?" Let yourself dream and tap into your deepest desires of what you want in life and why so you will set yourself up for success.

CHAPTER 5

ELIMINATE YOUR EXCUSES

The choices you make in your 40s will set you up for either a lifetime of feeling healthy, fit, and able to enjoy and experience more in life into your 50s, 60s, 70s, and beyond, or you'll spend these years feeling weaker, finding things harder to do, and becoming bogged down with injuries and health consequences. There are two very distinct paths as women turn 40.

It is too late in the game to keep making excuses and put off taking care of yourself. The time to start is now. Someday is today. Now is the time to build your team of support. Now is the time to learn how to make time and stop making excuses. Now is the time to unlock your ability to take control. Now is the time to be real with yourself about the changes that need to be made. Change is not easy; however, if you want more energy, health, and vitality, it is necessary.

A lifetime of programming yourself that you "can't" is about to get rewired to instead ask "how can I?" Realize that from a young age you may have been told you can't. You may have heard these statements before:

- You can't do a chin-up. Girls don't do chin-ups.
- You can't do a full push-up. Girls can do push-ups only from their knees.
- You can't lift too much weight. You'll hurt yourself.
- You can't run. Have you always told yourself that you're not a runner? You are if you want to be.
- You can't get in shape as you get older. Why not?

In the last chapter, you set some powerful goals and action steps for yourself. This chapter is about the most powerful piece of you accomplishing those goals, and that is getting your mind believing you can.

First, you need to overcome the excuses you hear. When these come up, you need an answer to overcome them. Don't worry, we have heard every excuse in the book and won't miss any. This chapter will leave you with no more excuses and ready to take action! It's not too late to age strong!

IDENTIFY YOUR PERSONAL EXCUSES

The following three barriers are the most common reasons women don't prioritize their strength training and personal goals. Which excuse or excuses have been your go-to?

I Don't Have Time

To shift how you think about time, start to think of time as space. Every one of us has the same allotted time or space—24 hours—in a day. We need to sleep 8 of those hours, which leaves 16 hours. If you work a full-time job five days a week, that takes eight hours of each work day, leaving you eight hours left per weekday and more on weekends. What are you prioritizing in those eight hours? Your family? Your friends? Your hobbies? Your health? Dedicating just one of those hours to your health every day is all you need. Spend an hour lifting weights, performing the Metabolic Cardio program in this book, or using a recovery strategy. Do this each day, and over time you will benefit in ways you never dreamed possible. You have the time (space). You have to decide you're worth carving out that space for yourself—and you are. The best part is that by giving yourself this one hour dedicated to your health, you'll have more to bring to the rest of the hours of your day, including energy for your family and friends.

I'm Too Tired

Fatigue can become an easy cycle to get into, especially if you've entered perimenopause and menopause. A lack of energy leads to consuming quick-energy foods higher in sugar, but that ends in an energy crash and not getting a restful sleep most nights, leaving you with no energy to work out. The fastest way to break this cycle is to work out. Working out will help you feel better, have more energy, and be less likely to grab quick-energy foods. You'll sleep better. Commit to showing up to work out, even if you're tired, and do what you can. We call these *clock-in workouts*. Not every workout is going to be a personal record–setting workout. Some are simply clock-in workouts. As you enter your 40s, think of your workout as non-negotiable. Many clients have shared they think of working out as their jobs, especially once they are retired. They have to do it.

I'm in Perimenopause or Menopause and My Hormones Are All Over the Place

Perimenopause or menopause can cause symptoms that make it feel impossible to prioritize working out and eating right. In the next chapter, I'll provide more detail about the cascade of hormonal fluctuations and symptoms you could be dealing with. Hormones are powerful. Take control of two aspects of your life—your workouts and your eating—to feel your best as you transition through perimenopause and menopause. To build lean muscle tissue, make strength training a priority. Eat foods that keep you fueled with the nutrients your body needs to feel your best and keep your blood sugar stable. Make working out a part of your prescription to get through the transition the best version of yourself you can. At no other time in your life has it been as important for you to take care of yourself as right now. Make sleeping, fueling your body with high-quality nutrition, managing stress, and exercising your priority.

GET OUT OF YOUR COMFORT ZONE

Now that you've overcome every excuse and will start to recognize when you are making them, it's time to start to shake things up. It's so easy as we get older to stay comfortable. Over time, staying comfortable means we miss out on progress, we miss out on experiences, and we miss out on growth.

When was the last time you pushed your mind and body beyond what it is already used to? Many women have a hard time doing this. I've seen that, when left on their own, women lift less weight than they are capable of. Learning to push beyond your comfort zone is a huge part of the success of this program. During this program, you'll be learning to grind out one last rep and that grunting to lift the heavier weight once in a while is OK and may be necessary to gain strength and feel fit.

I'm not saying women are averse to hard work. But it is rare to see a woman truly challenging herself in the weight room, especially as she ages. For some reason, in the weight room, women pick up the light dumbbells and do the exact opposite of what they need to develop the muscle to look and feel the way they want. Women have a higher pain tolerance than men; they just need to learn to apply it in the weight room.

Being around other women who are ready to push themselves, making an effort beyond what most women make, and realizing what's possible

Spotlight on Janelle Mault

Member since 2005

How old were you when you started strength training, and how old are you now?

I was in my 30s when I hired a personal trainer and then eventually joined Results Fitness when I was 36. I'm now 54 years old.

Why did you decide to make strength training a priority?

After having a baby, it was taking me a lot longer to look and feel the way I wanted to. With my primary goal as weight loss, I hired a personal trainer, and she recommended I strength train. We did mostly seated machines, but it got me started until I found Results Fitness, where my strength training really stepped up as a priority.

What was your experience going through perimenopause and menopause?

I had a hysterectomy at 35 years old, so I didn't have the obvious symptom of my period stopping. But I'm pretty sure I've been in perimenopause with some dramatic symptoms, including night sweats, bitchiness, and joint inflammation—I've felt achy for the past couple years. I finally decided to see the doctor and started HRT two months ago because my estrogen levels had dropped dramatically. My symptoms are now much better.

What results did you get by prioritizing strength training?

Strength training has increased my self-confidence. I have much less doubt about what I can do, both physically and emotionally. I'm capable of doing so much more than I thought. After following a structured strength training program for four years, at 40 years old, I decided to really challenge myself and enter my first competitive powerlifting event when I deadlifted a record for 155 pounds (70 kg). After training consistently, 10 years later in my 50s, I deadlifted 358 pounds (162 kg)! As I've gotten older, I've become stronger! I can do things I never thought I could do. I not only won gold medals in powerlifting but also ran six half marathons. I never in my life would have dreamed that I'd be a gold medal–winning powerlifter and a six-time half-marathoner!

How many days a week do you lift weights?

Three days a week.

What have you found to work for your nutrition?

I keep it super simple with my focus each day on getting enough protein by having a protein source at every meal. I always eat breakfast and have a postworkout shake, and I enjoy no more than seven alcoholic beverages a week.

What do you recommend to someone who is in their 40s wanting to age strong?

Get started today. You will surprise yourself. It's not hard. People think it's hard, but it's not hard. If you're looking for something that will improve the way you look and feel, it's really not that hard. You have to choose your "hard" as you age. You either choose losing strength, feeling less functional, and losing your independence and the ability to say yes to life experiences, or you choose to make time to prioritize strength training, which will keep you young, healthy, and fit. It surprises me how few people do not choose to make strength training a priority. It's not hard.

is extremely powerful. If you do anything at this time in your life, find other women who are also ready to do whatever it takes to look and feel their absolute best despite being at "that time in their life," when it's easy to give up and blame it on hormones.

In our gym, women push themselves every workout beyond what their bodies are used to, challenging themselves to get stronger. Try a little harder or set a challenging goal to get better every day. You can't help but be swept up by the inspiring women around you.

Entering my 40s, I had fallen into my own excuse trap, heading down the road I never thought I would. Looking back at my fire jump picture from my first Spartan Race, I see there is quite a change in me!

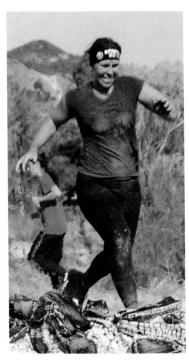 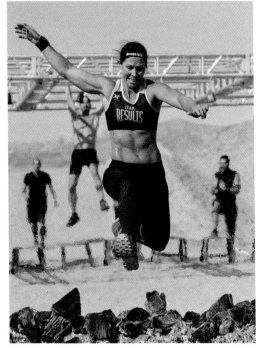

In the first picture, I'm timid, not sure of myself—even afraid—and 15 pounds (7 kg) heavier. In the second picture, I have an "I got this" badass Wonder Woman confidence going on.

Rachel Cosgrove

I think back to my first Spartan Race in 2015, which I *did not want to do*. I hadn't done a Spartan Race before and hadn't planned on it because it really didn't appeal to me. Doing something I wasn't comfortable with, challenging myself to overcome the mental barriers of an obstacle course race, pushed me in ways I never thought possible. Doing this race helped me to realize that even though I turned 40 that year, I could still challenge myself to learn new skills and have new experiences through a sport such as obstacle course racing. In fact, I stood on my first podium a couple of years later.

What is it about learning a new sport such as obstacle course racing, which I had no interest in before, that hooked me? It has to do with training for obstacles in the gym. I'm not just running to add more miles. Instead, I get to focus on getting stronger. Being strong gives you a real advantage in this event. Every race, I find something new to work on, whether it is an obstacle I haven't been able to get yet or a strategy to improve my performance. There are still obstacles I'm learning to do or to do better.

I love conquering obstacles that at one point felt impossible: *I'll never be able to climb a rope, I'm too heavy, I can't do those monkey bar obstacles.* Through practice, technique training, and strength gained from specific programming, I can now say the rope climb is no problem, and I have conquered most of the monkey bar obstacles. It's the best feeling ever to be able to swing my body across those bars like a kid again!

It's a privilege to line up next to other incredible women in the 40 to 49 age group who represent what being 40 looks like. At every race, I'm in awe of the women in my age group. They are a very small percentage of women who have not let age be an excuse for pushing themselves competitively.

You can't be afraid to approach near failure in your workouts. If every repetition and set is easy for you, you aren't applying a stimulus that will create any change. If you keep doing what you can already do, you'll keep having what you already have.

As you gain strength and confidence in your ability to use that strength, don't be afraid to try something new! Learn a new skill, sign up for a new adventure, or try something for the first time!

CONCLUSION

There are two distinct paths as you turn 40 and head into your 50s and 60s. You either can follow a road to losing strength, fitness, and independence or decide to actively work on building strength, power, balance, and stability to be able to stay active and independent and able to take care of yourself as you age strong.

CHAPTER 6

MANAGE MENOPAUSE

Being a woman in your 40s, 50s, and 60s means you're either approaching perimenopause, in perimenopause, have reached menopause, or have transitioned through menopause to officially be in postmenopause after one year of no periods. In this chapter, we will discuss the complex topic of hormones, something we as women have been experiencing fluctuations with and therefore symptoms from throughout our adult lives. I hope to simplify the complex topic of hormones to help you understand more about your own hormones and body while becoming aware of the individual differences and what you can control.

The list of symptoms that comes with perimenopause and menopause is daunting. Doctors have written many books covering this topic in depth. I'm not a doctor. The information you'll find in this chapter is gleaned from working with hundreds of women who have trained from their 40s through their 50s into their 60s and even 70s, along with studying and learning everything I can and of course my own personal experience as a woman. It's important to work closely with a doctor you trust. I'll share what I tell all my clients who have gone through or are going through perimenopause and menopause: Control what you can. This includes the following three things:

1. *Lift weights and build muscle.* You can gain strength and manage your body composition through the hormonal cycles of perimenopause and menopause. Strength training can help balance hormonal fluctuations. Follow the program in this book through this time, and you'll feel in control and more in balance.

2. *Fuel your body with healthy food to keep your blood sugar stable.* That will help keep your hormones stable. Following the nutrition advice in this book will help you to feel energized and strong.

3. *Manage stress.* Working out can really help with this, along with all the recovery strategies I'll be sharing, from breathing techniques to good sleeping habits.

ROLE OF HORMONES

Hormones are powerful, and we need to give ourselves grace as we navigate their ups and downs. This is about getting in tune with your body and learning what works for you and what doesn't and understanding how your body responds to different things.

Hormones are very complex, and they never work in isolation. One hormone fluctuating will send a cascade of other hormones into a cycle, like a domino effect in our body. The list of symptoms from these fluctuations as you go through menopause can be overwhelming. Some of the most common I've heard include feeling angry and irritable, noticing ankles or feet swelling, anxiety, back pain, bloating, depression, facial hair, fatigue, psychological feelings, fuzzy thinking, hair loss or thinning, headaches, adult acne, exacerbated allergies, heart palpitations, hot flashes, insomnia, joint pain, leg cramps, menstrual cycle irregularities, migraines, memory problems, mood swings, night sweats, panic attacks, and weight gain. With all that happening, no wonder you might be feeling stressed out and want to give up! Working out might be the last thing you want to do when you're not getting a good night's sleep.

A client first started to notice perimenopause symptoms in her early 40s before she became a member of Results Fitness. The first sign was when she suddenly couldn't multitask as well. As a schoolteacher, this became very difficult to manage. Shortly after that, her periods started to become sporadic and more symptoms started to pile on—high blood pressure; really bad hot flashes; itching, especially her ankles; joint pain, including inflammation in her knees; 20-pound (9 kg) weight gain and developing the "meno-apron" of fat that so many women experience; loss of strength; memory loss; increased anxiety and paranoia; and even a diabetes diagnosis. She tried managing her symptoms with medications for blood pressure, anxiety, and diabetes. I have no doubt she was experiencing a cascade of a hormonal domino effect. She moved from no medications to sudden, dramatic symptoms and necessary medications in a short time.

Midlife midsection, meno-pot belly, and *meno-apron* are examples of the not-so-nice names women give the belly fat that might never have been an issue before they entered perimenopause and menopause. Step one: End the negative self- talk! If you keep talking about yourself that way, it will be hard to ever overcome that negative mental dialogue. I even had a client say to me recently, "I have extra lard!" I quickly corrected her and said we don't use the word *lard* when you're talking about your beautiful, strong body. If you want to say it's "some extra stored energy," I'm OK with that.

I love the recent movement of women accepting themselves the way they are and no longer having negative self-talk. Talking negatively about your own body is self-destructive and affects you at a level you don't realize, keeping you from feeling your best. I always say, "The only perfect body is the one you woke up in!" There are many things we can't control, but one thing you can control is the things you say to yourself. Be nice.

I also understand not wanting to ignore an area of your body that doesn't look or feel the way it used to. It's OK to want to make changes, like I did as I entered my 40s and realized my body fat had reached over 30 percent. You can make changes without beating yourself up.

Let's talk about a few things to prioritize as you head into this time in your life so you can avoid a layer of abdominal fat being stored on your midsection:

- Manage your stress. Stress increases cortisol, which increases belly fat in women, as shown in a research study of 59 healthy premenopausal women (Epel et al. 2000).
- Get eight hours of sleep. People who get enough sleep have less visceral abdominal fat (discussed in chapter 3).
- Eliminate sugar. If sugar is your weakness, now is a really good time to change your habit of reaching for the sugar. Sugar can be a main culprit of so many of the cascading domino of hormonal symptoms that can be avoided.
- Eliminate alcohol, which is directly correlated with fat accumulation on the belly. People refer to it as a *beer belly* for a reason.
- Strength train to boost your muscle mass, metabolism, and the hormones that will keep you lean and strong. We'll cover this more in the rest of the chapter.

UNDERSTANDING HORMONES

In this book, to help you age strong, I'm going to discuss a few very specific hormones and how they interact with each other. It can feel like they are working against you and your goals, so I will also give you specific strategies to avoid dramatic symptoms. We will discuss our sex hormones, thyroid hormones, growth hormone, cortisol, and the hormones that regulate blood sugar.

Let's go through each hormone, what it does, and why fluctuations can cause symptoms. I'll cover the elements you can control to keep them as stable as possible. We will go through this list of hormones, starting from the bottom, or the base, of the column (figure 6.1) and working our way up. Everything underneath affects everything above.

Let's start at the base of the column. First, we will look at the sex hormones affected by perimenopause and menopause.

Testosterone

The first hormone, testosterone, is usually discussed when talking about male hormones, but it also plays a key role for women. Having enough testosterone increases lean muscle mass (so important as we go through menopause), decreases fat, and increases libido. Sometimes called our "mojo" hormone, levels of testosterone decline as we age. The changes are not as dramatic as with estrogen and progesterone levels during the menopause transition; instead, testosterone gradually decreases year after year.

You can control the following:

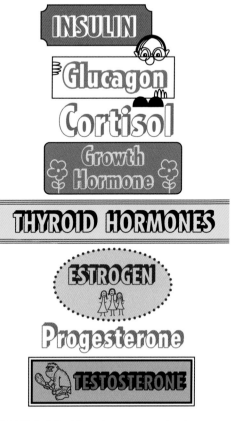

FIGURE 6.1   Your hormone stack.
Results Fitness

- Perform high-intensity exercise such as strength training and interval training. A study showed significant increases in testosterone after 15 weeks of resistance training in postmenopausal women (Ward et al. 2020).

- Consume more protein, including BCAAs from whey protein, to increase muscle protein synthesis.

- Lose body fat. A study showed that more body fat equals more estrogen, which means less testosterone (Janssen et al. 2010).

- The effects of zinc and magnesium supplements are mixed in the research, but some studies show supplementing increases free and total testosterone levels (Cinar et al. 2011).

- Consider a vitamin D supplement. Researchers observed a positive correlation between vitamin D levels and total testosterone levels in non-obese women (Masjedi et al. 2019).

- Reduce stress. High cortisol (the stress hormone) means lower testosterone levels according to the research (Kraemer et al. 2020).

- Eat healthy fats. Research shows a diet with less than 40 percent of calories from fat decreases testosterone in women (Ingram et al. 1987).

Spotlight on Lisa Clyde

Member since 2011

How old were you when you started strength training, and how old are you now?

I was 45 years old when I joined Results Fitness and started my first structured strength training program, and I'm now 58 years old. Before that, I was active and thought I was in pretty good shape.

Why did you decide to make strength training a priority?

I was going through a divorce and knew I needed to do something for myself. The gym became my safe place when I was going through my divorce. First, I did a short-term trial and thought it was too expensive. Then I realized I was worth it, and this needed to be a priority for me. I was 125 pounds (57 kg) when I joined, and in the first 6 months, I gained 15 pounds (7 kg) of lean body mass. I weighed more and looked so much better. I learned that being skinny didn't mean I was fit. As a dental hygienist, I had known patients who had suffered bad falls and bone breaks as they got older and saw them end up in and out of the hospital. I also realized I wanted to strength train to keep myself from ever getting osteoporosis.

What was your experience going through peri-menopause and menopause?

I started having symptoms when I was 51 years old, mainly feelings of anxiety I had never experienced before. When I saw my doctor, he asked me if I worked out and told me to increase my workouts from three times a week to five times a week. I started to connect that working out was the only way to get rid of the anxiety. Because of the anxiety, my habit of drinking wine had started to ramp up during menopause, until I realized it wasn't helping and was actually fueling my anxiety. I completely gave up wine and replaced it with working out more often as my remedy for my menopausal mood swings. My blood tests over the course of a year showed my estrogen dropping from 771 to 75! No wonder I was having symptoms. I remember driving home one night from work and calling my daughter, upset and bawling that I wasn't a good mother (which wasn't true), and my daughter said, "Go to the gym and work out and then we can talk." My family had even started to realize that working out balanced out my moods and was the answer to keeping Mom happy and feeling good. "Have you been to the gym yet today?" became their question anytime I seemed extra anxious or moody, and they were usually right. I just needed a good workout.

What results did you get by prioritizing strength training?

Besides managing my anxiety, I became strong for the first time in my life. I never had a weight problem, but I was skinny, not fit. I got hooked on feeling strong and loved it, realizing that the number on the scale didn't tell me the whole story. Gaining muscle was a very good thing. I

(continued)

(continued)

have accomplished more than I ever would have dreamed of, becoming an athlete in my 40s and 50s. I've now completed eight Spartan races and two half marathons. I'm proud of having a shapely, strong butt for the first time in my life. I love looking and feeling fit. Working out helped me through my divorce. Coming to the gym to work on myself and forget about everything going on in my life with the divorce kept me sane and got me through it.

How many days a week do you lift weights?

Five days a week during menopause, now three or four days a week.

What have you found to work for your nutrition?

After eliminating alcohol during menopause, I've decided to continue to not drink, realizing it wasn't giving me anything that I want to bring back and isn't good for me. Over the years, I've also learned how to eat to lose fat and not muscle. What works for me is five ounces of protein at each meal with some vegetables and a good fat, along with adding in some rice or quinoa for dinner. I eat only two meals a day—a big lunch and a big dinner—plus my postworkout shake. I've never been a breakfast person.

What do you recommend to someone who is in their 40s wanting to age strong?

Find a gym where you have a coach, a customized program, and a community. Getting the proper programming is game-changing and makes a big difference, as does accountability on your nutrition and a community of people you connect with. Finding people who are really like-minded and meeting some of my best friends at the gym has been life-changing. Don't be afraid to invest in yourself. Make your health and fitness a priority in your budget. When I got re-married, paying for my gym membership was a non-negotiable in our budget as a couple.

What's next?

I'll continue to compete and race. I want to be able to do everything I can do as long as I can do it. I already have friends in their 60s who think they can't do stuff. I know they could if they chose to put the effort in to work out, start gaining strength, and keep themselves fit and strong. I want to avoid saying "I can't" for as long as possible.

Progesterone

Progesterone and estrogen are the primary hormones that drop off during menopause, creating many of the dramatic symptoms women experience. You need a balance of these hormones to feel good. Progesterone is a potent fat burner, aids in libido, thins the uterine lining, regulates the menstrual cycle, and is key for fertilization and pregnancy. A decrease in progesterone can lead to the symptoms of menopause many women experience.

Besides working closely with your doctor to help you navigate your specific hormone fluctuations and decide whether hormone replacement therapy (HRT) is something you should do, you can take other actions to make a difference.

You can control the following:

- Consume vitamin B6, either through food or supplementation. Vitamin B6 has been shown to help in the production of progesterone (Lee 2020). If you are deficient, your body's production of progesterone could dramatically decrease. Vitamin B6 also helps the liver to properly break down estrogen, which prevents a hormonal imbalance caused by excess estrogen. Make sure your body has plenty of vitamin B6 by taking a high-quality multivitamin and eating foods rich in vitamin B6, including potatoes, beans, spinach, bananas, seafood, poultry, red meat, whole grains, and walnuts.

- Eliminate or decrease alcohol intake to allow your liver to do its job of breaking down estrogen and keeping your hormones in balance. The liver is where your hormones are processed.

Estrogen

Estrogen levels drop during menopause, causing many symptoms. Estrogen is an anabolic hormone, meaning it tells your body to grow. High estrogen can mean more subcutaneous fat distribution, giving us our baby-bearing hips necessary for childbirth. As we enter menopause, we no longer need to be able to bear children, so estrogen drops. This can be one of the reasons your body shape will change from having hips and thighs to suddenly having more fat on your belly than before. Another important role of estrogen is as an anti-cortisol hormone; higher estrogen helps keep cortisol, the stress hormone, in balance. As estrogen levels decrease, you'll notice increased frequency of mood swings and cravings; decreased levels of serotonin, dopamine, and gamma-aminobutyric acid (GABA); distribution of fat on belly; and hot flashes.

You can control the following:

- Decrease environmental estrogens. Plastics, processed dairy, and processed meats have chemicals that mimic or antagonize the natural estrogen your body produces, which, according to a study published in *Environmental Health Perspectives,* is the most common form of hormone disruption (Yang et al. 2011).

- Consume flaxseeds, which can help balance estrogen by binding to estrogen in the intestine (Brooks et al. 2004).

- Eat a high-fiber diet. Having regular bowel movements decreases estrogen absorption in the colon.

Thyroid Hormones

The thyroid is a regulator, controlling many of the body's most important functions and affecting nearly every organ. Think of the thyroid as a thermostat that keeps the body at homeostasis by making hormones that control the way the body uses energy. This is what the thyroid is responsible for:

- Regulating body temperature. The thyroid produces hormones that dilate the blood vessels and affect how much heat leaves the body.
- Regulating metabolism. The thyroid changes the basal metabolic rate by increasing or decreasing oxygen consumption, respiration, and body temperature.
- Regulating energy. The thyroid influences key metabolic pathways through the brain, white fat, brown fat, muscle, liver, and the pancreas.

You can control the following:

- Avoid soy, which has been shown to inhibit the thyroid gland and increase thyroid stimulating hormone (TSH) after consumption (Otun et al. 2019).
- Manage stress to maintain good adrenal health.
- Maintain balanced insulin levels by eating protein, good fats, and fruits and vegetables throughout the day.
- Eliminate aspartame, which appeared to be the culprit in a study on the development of Hashimoto's thyroiditis (Sachmechi et al. 2018).
- Perform intense exercise, which has been shown to increase thyroid hormones. Exercise performed at 70 percent of max heart rate caused an increase in thyroid hormones (Ciloglu et al. 2005). However, avoid overtraining, which can put you into adrenal and thyroid fatigue.

Growth Hormone

Growth hormone controls everything from bone to muscles to our height and helps to regulate sugar and fat metabolism, body composition, and body fluids. Growth hormone peaks when we're young, making it easier to build muscle and maintain a healthy body composition. As we age, growth hormone declines. Growth hormone does these tasks:

- Mobilizes free fatty acids
- Decreases glucose uptake (when insulin is high, growth hormone is low)

- Increases fat burned from the lower body
- Increases lean muscle growth

You can control the following:

- Perform intense exercise such as metabolic interval training, which has been shown to increase growth hormone (Wideman et al. 2002).
- Consume more protein and good fats.
- Engage in strength training.

Cortisol

Cortisol is a stress hormone, telling our body it is in flight-or-fight mode. Cortisol levels should be highest in the morning and lowest in the evening to make it easier to fall asleep. For many people, cortisol levels are flipped; they wake up tired and then experience a rise in cortisol through the day due to the daily fires that come up until they are lying awake at night, unable to sleep. Cortisol and melatonin are on opposite schedules; if cortisol is high, melatonin will be low, which does not help the sleeping situation. Cortisol tells the body it's under stress. It breaks down muscle when the body is in survival mode. Because of its actions when the body is under stress, cortisol is the number one pro-aging hormone. Research has linked high levels of cortisol to low levels of thyroid hormone (Walter et al. 2012). High levels of cortisol may lead to cravings for quick energy, especially sugar. Those who experience high levels of cortisol may find themselves tired in the morning but stressed and wired by the end of the day, making it difficult to sleep.

You can control the following:

- Take time to de-stress. Do something every day to decompress and lower your cortisol level. Deep breathing, meditation, or stretching may help.
- Take inventory of your "Tub o' Stress" to identify anything you can eliminate.
- Make your sleep a priority.
- Don't work out more than an hour at a time.
- Have a postworkout protein and carbohydrate shake. Cortisol will rise during your workout as muscle tissue breaks down and you stress your body. Consuming protein and carbohydrate postworkout will blunt the rise in cortisol. Research has shown that consuming a shake that includes protein and carbohydrate after your workout reduces cortisol and improves recovery (Bird et al. 2006).

Glucagon and Insulin

The last two hormones on the column relate to blood sugar regulation and food consumption. Insulin tells your body to store fat when your blood sugar is high. Insulin levels will rise, letting your body know there is excess that needs to be stored. Glucagon is opposite to insulin; it is released when it's time to burn fat stores and blunts insulin from storing fat.

You can control the following:

- Decrease your intake of processed foods, including foods high in sugar.
- Have protein with each meal.
- Eat fats with each meal.
- Eat throughout the day.

Other Hormones

These hormones also can be affected during perimenopause and menopause:

- **Serotonin** is our feel-good hormone. You can positively affect your levels of serotonin by exercising regularly.
- **Leptin** helps to manage metabolism, hunger, and energy. It's known as the satiety hormone. To keep this hormone in balance, do not restrict calories below your basal metabolic rate.
- **Ghrelin** is a hunger hormone; it can increase appetite and food intake and promote fat storage. By eating regularly, you can limit the effects of ghrelin.
- **Vitamin D** is starting to be thought of as a hormone. It strengthens the immune system and has a role in controlling blood pressure, may offer cancer protection, improves asthma, and help to prevent blood clots. You can maintain a healthy level of vitamin D by getting regular exposure to sunshine and supplementing if prescribed by your health care professional.

Make an appointment to get an annual physical with your doctor where they can check your hormone levels now to be able to compare as time goes on. It's a really good idea to start to build your relationship with your doctor so they know you, and you trust them.

Earlier, I shared a client's experience with the many symptoms she encountered. She started to get serious about her strength training. She had always been active and was even a Jazzercise instructor. In her 40s, she watched her mom decline after being diagnosed with breast

Should You Use Hormone Replacement Therapy (HRT)?

This is a question for your doctor; answering it is outside my scope of practice. What I will tell you is that you cannot out-hormone a lifestyle of no sleep; no exercise; too much sugar, alcohol, and processed foods; and high stress.

Adding hormone replacement therapy on top of poor lifestyle choices that are making it harder for your body to handle the changes isn't going to fill the gap of everything you can improve. Take care of your body by adding muscle mass through strength training two or three times a week, eating enough protein to recover, maintaining optimal hydration, consuming a diet high in fiber and low in processed foods and alcohol to help your body stay in balance, getting enough sleep, managing your stress, and taking a few supplements that help decrease inflammation and give your body what it needs. Are you doing all that and still feel the symptoms of menopause? Then definitely discuss HRT with your doctor.

Some clients go on HRT, and others get through menopause without it. A few started HRT after menopause as their hormones were still stabilizing. I'm not against using HRT and believe everybody is different with individual needs. If you are already doing everything you can to give your body what it needs to handle the fluctuating hormones of the transition and the symptoms are unbearable, then you definitely need to discuss HRT with your doctor.

cancer and was motivated to build strength as she aged. Despite having a tough time through menopause, she became very consistent with her strength training, lifting weights three days a week. Even though her strength gains may not have been as good as if she wasn't going through menopause, she made strength training a habit she will never give up and knows she'll be strong and ready for whatever life throws her way. If you haven't entered into perimenopause and menopause yet, now is the time to start your habit of lifting weights, building strength, and making yourself a priority.

CONCLUSION

Managing changing hormones can be a frustrating piece of the puzzle as we age. We may sometimes feel like nothing is under our control and our own body is working against us. Instead, focus on the actions you can control to help your body function as optimally as possible, keeping hormone fluctuations to a minimum to avoid dramatic symptoms. By following the action steps in this chapter, you'll be able to coast through perimenopause and menopause much easier!

CHAPTER 7

RECORD YOUR PROGRESS

It is important to record your progress and keep track of where you are in relation to where you are going. After the goal-setting chapter, where you decided what your powerful goals are, you'll need a way to measure whether you're getting there.

Think like a scientist as you approach your fitness programming, nutrition, recovery, and every effort you're putting in to feel your absolute best as you age. It's simply an equation. Take the emotions out of it (hard, I know) and look at the data.

Everything you've done up until now in your lifetime has added up to your current result. The food you ate each day, the hours of sleep each night, the beverages you consumed, the stress you took on—each one is a line item on the spreadsheet adding up to your current health. Some are chipping away as liabilities, subtracting from your long-term health, and others are assets adding to your long-term health.

If you're feeling strong, fit, and healthy, then hopefully you've tracked what you've been doing so you can keep doing it. At Results Fitness, clients gave me their data to now share with you what works. We know because we kept track.

> What gets measured gets managed.
> Peter Drucker

If you want to change something (the way you feel, lose weight, be injured less often), you have to try something different from what you've been doing. Track it and see what result you get.

It's that simple. No emotion. No beating yourself up. Just X + Y = Z. Tracking it is key so you know what you did.

KEY INDICATORS TO TRACK

Let's start by checking where you currently are. What has your current lifestyle equation equaled? Consider tracking four key indicators every year to check in on how your progress is trending, starting now. These indicators are your blood markers, body composition, strength training volume, and progress toward being able to do something new. Let's look at each of these indicators in more detail.

Blood Tests

An annual physical is no longer optional as you enter your 40s. Establish a good relationship with your doctor and keep a history of your bloodwork on file to know what's normal for you and whether your blood markers are showing that you are getting healthier year after year, staying the same, or heading in the wrong direction. Finding out sooner than later gives you the opportunity to do something about it. Change the equation!

Discuss with your doctor which basic blood tests you need to do every year. Depending on your health, family history, lifestyle, and other factors, you may need to do the following:

- A lipoprotein panel, including LDL (bad cholesterol), HDL (good cholesterol), and triglycerides
- A metabolic panel, including blood glucose, calcium, electrolytes, kidney, and liver function
- GGT (liver enzyme)
- A complete blood count (CBC) that measures red blood cells, white blood cells, and platelets
- Hemoglobin A1c
- C-reactive protein
- Homocysteine
- Uric acid
- Insulin
- Vitamin D3
- An iron panel, including serum iron, ferritin, TIBC, and percent of iron saturation
- A thyroid panel, including TSH, free T3 and T3 total, free T4 and T4 total, reverse T3, and thyroid antibodies
- A hormone profile, including estrogen, estradiol, DHEA-S, progesterone, and testosterone (both total and free)

Body Composition

For many people, the scale is the indicator of "Oh my God, I hit THAT number and need to do something!" There has been research that indicates weighing yourself daily does equal maintaining weight loss long term (Burke, Wang, and Sevick 2011; Linde et al. 2005; Vanwormer et al. 2008; Welsh et al. 2009). However, as you start to make strength training a priority, the scale is not going to be your best measure of your body composition. Strength training will build muscle (which we want) and even bone (which we especially want as we age), and muscle and bone do weigh something. Even the glycogen you store in your muscles to use for fuel during your workouts will add to that scale number.

As you become a workout goddess, you'll no longer use the scale as your most accurate measurement. You can get on it daily if you like to collect the data. That's all it is—it's just data. It'll tell you if last night's dinner had extra sodium and made you more bloated so you temporarily weigh more or if the days after you work out you seem to be heavier because you're storing more glycogen. If you haven't gone number 2 yet, guess what? The number is also higher. This doesn't mean you've gained fat.

You're learning a lot about your body and how it works. Bottom line: If you're going to get on the scale regularly, please take what it tells you as an educated scientist as simply data. It's not going to ruin your day or tell you you're fat. It's not going to cause binge eating or a starvation diet or send you into a depression. It's an inanimate metal object that is telling you at that moment what you weigh. That's all.

In addition, doctors will often use body mass index (BMI), which brings height into the equation as simply a measure of the relationship between your height and your weight. This could be an accurate measurement for someone who is sedentary, along with looking at the population on average telling us who has higher body fat according to their BMI and therefore a higher risk of disease. For the small percentage (unfortunately) of people who strength train, BMI is not an accurate measurement of your health.

Measuring Body Composition

A more accurate way to assess your body composition is to use a body composition analyzer, which will tell you more information about what your weight is made up of and if you are gaining weight that is the good stuff. If it is, fantastic! We want that kind of weight! Adding muscle weight is an asset to our long-term health.

There are many ways to analyze body composition, and some are easier than others. Here are a few.

• **Inbody Body Composition Analyzer.** We've found this to be the most accurate and convenient. The Inbody analyzer uses bioelectrical impedance (BIA) technology to gauge your muscle, fat, and water composition. We have one at Results Fitness and recommend our clients use it at least once a month. When you use it to measure, you'll be able to check trends of what is actually happening with your progress, especially if you're putting in extra effort. Because it does not require you to dunk under water or do anything drastic, it's easy to use often to check in. To get the most accurate measurement, have an empty stomach, be hydrated (no alcohol the night before), and avoid doing it right before or during your menstrual cycle. While handheld BIA machines can be somewhat accurate if you use them under the same conditions every time, it's more likely that readings will fluctuate than if you use a medical-grade analyzer like Inbody.

• **Hydrostatic weighing.** In college, as an exercise and health minor with a physiology degree, I had access to a hydrostatic weighing scale. We had to test each other, getting our hydrostatic weight, and then use body fat calipers to see how close we would get. Using a hydrostatic scale isn't convenient for most people unless you're a college student with access to one anytime you'd like. It is a giant tank of water with a scale inside. You enter the tank and sit on the scale, exhaling all the air you can out of your lungs to get your weight under water. Since fat floats and muscle sinks, you'll find out what you weigh under water. That number is equal to your lean body mass, and the difference of your weight tells you how many pounds of fat you are carrying. This is one of the most accurate ways to find out your body composition but also the most inconvenient.

• **Bodyfat calipers.** If you are working with a professional coach trained to use body fat calipers, this can also be a very accurate measurement and is how we measured our clients for years before we found the Inbody machine. You'll have the fat in four areas of your body pinched by a caliper and plugged into an equation to calculate your body fat percentage. It's most accurate if the same person conducts the test every time. One unpleasant aspect of using calipers is that nobody likes to have their fat pinched, so you may not be comfortable subjecting yourself to the assessment.

• **How your clothing fits.** This is my favorite method of assessing body composition changes. The scale could stay the same or go up, but if your tight pair of jeans are getting looser, you know you're gaining muscle and losing fat. The biggest breakthrough for many of our clients is when I have them take a break from using a scale and stop looking at that number and instead use a pair of pants as their measurement. We've consistently seen that our clients on average will lose only 4 pounds (2 kg) on the scale while dropping two whole clothing sizes in the first 8 to 12 weeks of training because they're gaining muscle and losing fat, changing their composition.

Interpreting Body Composition Measurements

According to the *American Journal of Clinical Nutrition* (Gallagher et al. 2000), women aged 40 to 59 with a body fat percentage over 33 percent are considered unhealthy. If you measure and find that your body fat percentage is 33 percent or more, remember that this is data. Everything you've been doing added up to this result. We need to make changes to get a different result, which is why you're reading this book. Having 20 to 33 percent body fat will get you into the healthy range.

Remember that changing your body composition is not only an indicator that you are losing body fat. For many women over 40, gaining muscle is just as, if not more, important to changing their body composition. If you are 150 pounds (68 kg) and have 50 pounds (23 kg) of fat with the other 100 pounds (45 kg) of lean body mass—which is everything other than fat (muscle, water, bone, organs)—then you have 33 percent body fat. If you gain just 5 pounds (2 kg) of muscle during this program to now weigh 155 pounds (70 kg) and lose 5 pounds (2 kg) of fat (which will be much easier to do and maintain with your new muscle), you'll be under 30 percent and in a healthy range.

Please do not get obsessed with the numbers and instead remember to treat it as data. If you're working hard, doing a ton of cardio, and watching what you're eating yet trending in the wrong the direction—gaining fat and losing muscle—you want to know that so that you can take a different approach like the one in this book to prioritize strength training and fuel your body with the food it needs to be healthy and strong.

Progress During Workouts

Tracking your workouts will give you the data to know whether you are getting stronger and improving your fitness. Through the programs in this book, you'll progress through exercises, and as a check-in at the end of each phase, you'll do a set of as many as you can get to see if you're lifting close to your ability. With each workout, you should be lifting more weight and doing more volume of work.

To make sure you are adding more volume, you'll want to track what you lift each workout and throughout each phase so you know the percentage increase you're making in volume (reps × sets × load) and intensity (your heart rate during your metabolic interval sessions).

Your Ability to Do Something

Having external accountability is *everything*. Most people need it. We discussed this in depth in the chapter on goal setting. This can be in the form of a race, a competition, or simply an exercise in the gym you want to conquer. Being able to perform your first push-up or chin-up or deadlift your body weight is a great indicator of your progress. I recommend having something you're training for every three or four months at least. Find a race or event and get registered. Nothing will motivate you more to not miss a workout!

I love to test myself on the race course. Nothing pushes me like crossing a start line to try to get to the finish line as fast as I can. I'm competing against the other women in my age group, but I'm also competing against myself.

Spotlight on Sharon Tyler

Member since 2006

How old were you when you started strength training, and how old are you now?

I was 44 years old when I started, and I just turned 61 years old.

Why did you decide to start making strength training a priority?

By my mid 40s I had gained 25 pounds (11 kg) and was having a hard time losing it for 10 years. Then my mom was diagnosed with osteoporosis, which also became a motivation. After a bone scan, I found out I was also at high risk. I wanted to lose weight and reduce that risk.

What was your experience going through perimenopause and menopause?

By the time I entered premenopause, I had already started strength training and was starting to lose fat gradually. The pounds were slow to come off, but I focused on the process of building muscle to avoid getting discouraged. I was determined to get through menopause without going on hormone replacement therapy, despite low energy and hot flashes. I focused on the things I could control, such as exercise, nutrition, and sleep. Postmenopause and now down in weight, I'm holding some body fat differently, such as a thicker middle, but I also know it would be even more pronounced if I hadn't stuck to my strength training.

What results did you get by prioritizing strength training?

By combining strength training with changes in my nutrition and sleep, I came through menopause with relative ease. I ended up getting into the best shape of my life in my 50s. Now in my 60s, I retired from my corporate career and decided to get a part-time job at Trader Joe's, where the work is very physically demanding. I'm able to meet the physical demands of the job due to my years of strength training.

How many days a week do you lift weights?

Twice a week.

What have you found to work for your nutrition?

I track my food and make sure I get at least 100 grams of protein every day. I enjoy myself, splurging without guilt one or two times a week. I always eat breakfast and rarely drink alcohol. My focus has shifted from losing weight to focus on longevity. I make sure I'm fueling my body with fruits and vegetables, eating a rainbow of foods, and realizing how powerful food can be to my well-being. You truly are what you eat. I've realized that instead of quick fixes (what I was looking for when I first started), it's better to have gradual changes over time. They build on each other and have set me up for long-term success with my health and fitness as I age strong.

What do you recommend to someone who is in their 40s wanting to age strong?

> Think about what your goals are. How do you want to live in your 50s and 60s? Gradually start making changes instead of expecting a quick fix. Create motivation for yourself by making the commitment to be consistent, no matter what. People think I'm naturally motivated, and I'm not. Train yourself to work out, even when you don't feel like it. You won't always feel motivated. You'll build that habit, just like building a muscle along the way. Action creates motivation. I think of working out as my job. You'll struggle with transforming yourself if you depend on always being motivated. It's a choice.

WRITE IT DOWN

Why is it important to make frequent progress checks in these areas? First, it will help motivate you. If you check on your progress regularly, you'll know if your efforts are helping you move in the direction you want to go. If you wait too long between check-ins, you may be heading in the wrong direction and not realize it. The more often you do them, the less pressure there is on each one. If you are racing a 5K once a month and have one slow performance, there's always next month, and since you tracked what you did, you'll realize that not getting enough sleep the week before equaled a slower performance. Next time, sleep will be a priority!

Second, as time goes by and life veers in different directions, it is easy for things to start to slip. The things you know make you feel good get put on the back burner for a day, a week, a whole month, and the "degree of slippage" can easily get completely off track over time. By committing to checking in regularly to these indicators, you'll catch yourself before you get too far off track. Knowing you'll be checking in regularly will already keep your subconscious prioritizing the things that will keep you moving in the right direction. Commit now to how often you'll check in on these indicators and set the next date after you do your initial check-in, and you'll catch yourself before you start to slack.

Also, by checking your progress, you'll know if you've hit a plateau and are staying the same. If you aren't tracking what you're lifting or how much progress you're making, you won't know that it's time to make a change. Your body has adjusted to your current program, and you need to switch things up! Nothing works forever. Our bodies are too smart for that. You'll need to continually push, change, and put new demands on your body if you want to keep making progress.

Progress is not always linear. By checking often, you'll be able to see the trends rather than put pressure on a single measurement every once

AGE STRONG HABIT TRACKER FORM

For the 16 weeks you're following the program from this book, track your habits to start making some serious changes and coast through feeling strong in your 40s, 50s, 60s, and beyond! Our clients get a nightly text with these same habit tracker items to make note of each night.

		WEEK							
Habit	**Goal**	**1**	**2**	**3**	**4**	**5**	**6**	**7**	**8**
Strength training	2-3 times per week								
Hydration	0.5 × body weight per day								
Breakfast	Daily								
Protein intake	1 g per pound of lean body mass per day								
Vegetable intake	3-5 servings daily								
Fiber intake	25 g per day								
Alcohol intake	Less than 2 servings per day								
Supplements	Four core daily								
Recovery	Daily								
De-stress	1 time per day (minimum)								
Sleep	7-8 hr per night								
Notes									

		WEEK							
Habit	**Goal**	**9**	**10**	**11**	**12**	**13**	**14**	**15**	**16**
Strength training	2-3 times per week								
Hydration	0.5 times body weight per day								
Breakfast	Daily								
Protein intake	1 g per pound of lean body mass per day								
Vegetable intake	3-5 servings daily								
Fiber intake	25 g per day								
Alcohol intake	Less than 2 servings per day								
Supplements	Four core daily								
Recovery	Daily								
De-stress	1 time per day (minimum)								
Sleep	7-8 hr per night								
Notes									

in a while. You're going to have weeks and months when stress is higher than normal or you weren't able to be as consistent and your progress will be affected. It's no big deal. We're in this for the long haul. Continuing to check in regularly will show you that you're trending in the right direction over time.

In addition to the longer-term outcome goal progress indicators, tracking your daily habits and focusing on your process goals (learn more about these in the chapter about setting goals) will help you to stay proactive by being consistent day after day.

To start tracking daily, do the following:

- A journal works great! This could be a pen-and-paper journal if you enjoy writing, or there are several apps and digital options now. Find a time daily when you can take 10 minutes to check in with yourself. Jot down in a journal the last 24 hours, including your workout, your nutrition, and how you're feeling, and include a measurement of gratitude in there too ("I'm grateful for") to not only focus on the progress you want to make but also realize how far you've come and what a great job you've done. Our clients get a digital journal texted to them each night, tracking their sleep, water consumption, protein servings, vegetable servings, alcohol servings, and a place to write a note about how the day went.

- If you're ready to get specific with your nutrition, it's a good idea to use a digital tracker to get an idea of how many calories you're eating and how much protein, carbs, and fat to get the data to be able to make a change if the result is not progressing. If you don't know what you're doing, it's hard to make a change.

CONCLUSION

At this point, I hope you're starting to think scientifically about this journey. It's easy to get emotional when it comes to your body, which is why it's important to check the data and see exactly where you are, how far you've come, and where you want to go. By checking in on your progress, you'll feel good about the efforts you're putting in to keep it up!

PART III

THE EXERCISES

CHAPTER 8

WARM-UP

First things first—let's warm up! Before we get into each phase, I want to introduce a dynamic warm-up, which will be how you start every training session to get your body ready. At this stage in the game, we cannot get away with jumping straight into a workout without warming up. To keep yourself injury-free and get the most out of your workouts, you have to include a thorough and dynamic warm-up such as the one described in this chapter.

This warm-up is more than a 10-minute walk on the treadmill. It's part of the workout, increasing your range of motion and flexibility, elevating your heart rate and body temperature, and getting your adrenaline flowing to stimulate your nervous system and increase blood flow to your muscles. We actually call it a RAMP, or range of motion, activation, and movement preparation. Perform this warm-up before you head into each workout. You can also perform it on a recovery day as movement to get your blood flowing and work on your range of motion.

Each phase of the warm-up will help you learn movement patterns, gain strength, and improve mobility. You'll be getting so strong that the moves initially part of your workout will eventually become your warm-up! Take your time going through each phase of these exercises as we train your body to move properly.

Every RAMP features exercises in these categories:

1. Self-massage (usually two to four areas)
2. Positional breathing reset
3. Hip mobility (usually three different ones)
4. Thoracic spine mobility
5. Ankle mobility
6. Combination of movements
7. Patterning (hip hinge)
8. Patterning (asymmetrical squat or lunge)
9. Patterning (symmetrical squat)
10. Movement skills
11. Neural activation

As you go through each phase of the RAMP, you can choose a different version of that category if the one programmed is too difficult.

SELF-MASSAGE

Using a foam roller before starting your workout will prepare muscles and reduce excess muscle tension by affecting the nervous system and improving blood flow. Go through the following movements to feel great heading into your workout.

> **PRO CUE:** Move slowly and purposefully while foam rolling. If you paid for a massage, you wouldn't want to have the massage therapist go as fast as possible, would you?

FOAM ROLL THE HIPS

Start with the hips and work your way out to the limbs.

Position

Sit on the foam roller. Cross one foot over the other and lean toward the hip of the crossed leg (figure 8.1).

Movement

Roll up and down on that hip, working your way around the entire gluteal muscle to find any hot spots. If you do find a dense or sore spot, stay there and breathe for a few seconds to get it to release. Repeat on the other side.

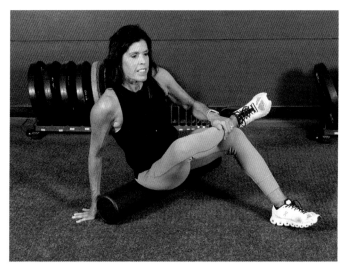

FIGURE 8.1   Foam roll the hips.

FOAM ROLL THE HAMSTRINGS

Work your way down the back of each leg.

Position

Sit on the foam roller with your legs straight out in front. Cross one leg over the other to increase the pressure. The bottom leg is the one getting rolled. Place your hands behind you on the floor for support (figure 8.2).

Movement

Roll up and down from just under the crease of your glutes to the knee. Repeat on the other side.

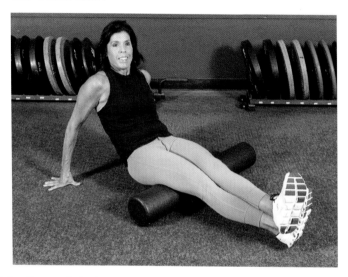

FIGURE 8.2   Foam roll the hamstrings.

FOAM ROLL THE CALVES

Hot spots in the calves are very common. Be prepared to spend some time releasing any tightness that will affect your ankle mobility and everything else up the posterior chain.

Position

Place your calf on the foam roller with your legs straight out in front. The foam roller will be under your knee. Cross one leg over the other to increase the pressure (figure 8.3). The bottom leg is the being rolled. Place your hands behind you on the floor for support.

Movement

Roll the calf from under the knee to the ankle, toes pointing straight up. Then turn the foot inward to hit a different part of the calf. Finally turn the foot outward while slowly rolling up and down across the calf. Repeat on the other side.

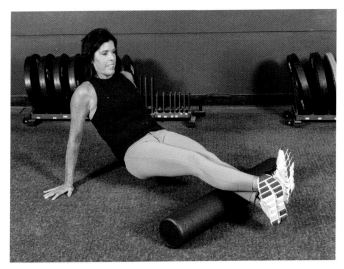

FIGURE 8.3   Foam roll the calves.

FOAM ROLL THE QUADRICEPS

Once you've rolled the back of your legs, flip over to hit the front of your legs.

Position

Lie face down with the foam roller underneath the tops of your thighs. Lean to one side with the other leg crossed over the back to increase pressure (figure 8.4).

Movement

Roll up and down from the hip to the knee. Repeat on the other side.

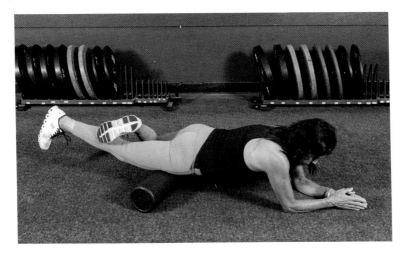

FIGURE 8.4 Foam roll the quadriceps.

FOAM ROLL THE ADDUCTORS

Move over to the insides of your legs to get the chronically tight adductor muscles.

Position

Lie face down with one leg externally rotated. Place the roller perpendicular to your bent leg on the inside of your thigh (figure 8.5). You are rolling the inner thigh area.

Movement

Roll from your groin to the inside of your knee. Repeat on the other side.

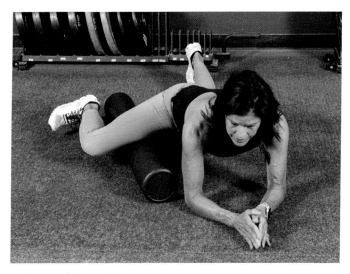

FIGURE 8.5   Foam roll the adductors.

FOAM ROLL THE LATS

The latissimus dorsi muscle group can create problems at the shoulder. It's important to keep the lats functioning optimally for the health of your shoulder joints.

Position

Lie on your side on the roller with your arm up so the roller is under your armpit (figure 8.6).

Movement

Roll from your armpit to the top of the hip, turning your body to hit different angles of the big muscle, the latissimus dorsi (lats). Repeat on the other side.

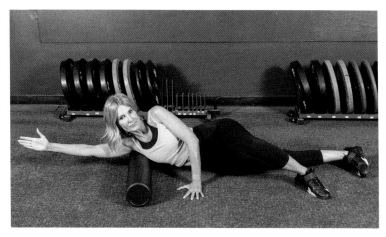

FIGURE 8.6   Foam roll the lats.

FOAM ROLL THE MID TO UPPER BACK

Rolling this area will stimulate your vagus nerve and prepare you to train. It's a perfect way to finish your foam rolling.

Position

Lie on the floor with the foam roller beneath your upper back and parallel to your shoulders. Place your hands behind your head to support your neck (figure 8.7).

Movement

With your elbows out, slowly roll your upper back up and down over the foam roller from your bra line to your shoulders and trapezius muscles.

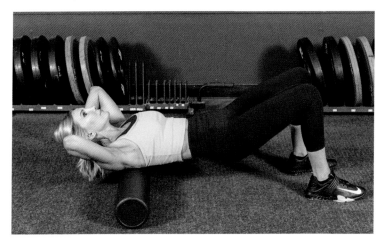

FIGURE 8.7 Foam roll the mid to upper back.

POSITIONAL BREATHING RESET

Many clients appreciate spending time to reset using a breathing drill. This positional breathing reset with help you recenter by restoring the body to a parasympathetic state. Some clients find themselves going back to do this exercise again throughout the day. Deep diaphragmatic breathing will bring your body in alignment with your core and prepare you to work properly.

POSITIONAL BREATHING RESET

Think of your core like a canister, as we discussed in chapter 1. Using your diaphragm to breathe will help align your canister.

Position

Lie on the floor in a comfortable position with your arms at your sides. Feel free to bend the knees so your feet are flat on the floor or put your feet against a wall to form a 90-degree angle. Or if you prefer, come into a child's pose: Sit back on your heels. Slowly bend forward to bring your forehead to the floor, keeping your stomach between your thighs and your buttocks as close to your heels as you can. You can put your hands next to your legs, palms up, or put them out in front of you, palms down.

Movement

Breathe in through the nose for 5 seconds; hold the breath for 3 seconds; and fully exhale through the mouth or nose for 5 seconds, releasing all the air. Hold for 3 seconds again before repeating. As you breathe in, think about the ribs moving outward and all the way around, expanding 360 degrees.

PRO CUE: Think of starting the breath low in the pelvis and visualize it moving outward and upward through your torso, as if you are filling up a pitcher of water.

HIP MOBILITY

Lacking hip mobility as we age is very common and can be one of the main reasons for low-back pain, along with other compensating movements affecting how well you can move. Performing exercises to improve hip mobility needs to be a priority for women over 40, starting with the warm-up to get the body moving properly for the workout.

HALF-KNEELING HIP FLEXOR MOBILITY

This stretch will create mobility in the hips, undoing tight hip flexors from a lot of sitting, walking, or running.

Position

Kneel on the knee of the hip you'll be stretching, the other leg bent at 90 degrees and the foot on the floor. Keep a tall posture. Place a towel or pad under the back knee for comfort if needed.

Movement

Maintain a tall posture while you tilt your hips under (figure 8.8). Imagine wearing a belt and tilting your imaginary belt buckle toward the ceiling as you slowly push your hips forward. Tighten your glutes as your hips move forward to increase the stretch. Keep your core and glutes engaged. Repeat on the other side.

PRO CUE: Think about "hiding" the lower ribs to keep the ribs and pelvis connected to make sure you are moving through the hip joint versus extending the lower back.

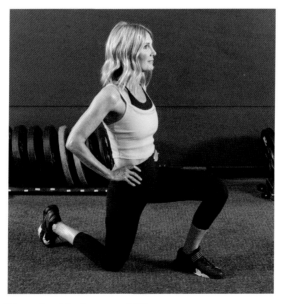

FIGURE 8.8   Half-kneeling hip flexor mobility.

WINDSHIELD WIPER 90/90 HIP STRETCH

This is a gentle mobility movement for the hip joint to improve mobility and release any tension in your lower back. You'll be moving through both internal rotation and external rotation of both hips.

Position

Sit on the floor with your arms out straight behind you for support. Bend both knees to 90 degrees.

Movement

Drop both knees to one side, putting one hip in internal rotation and the other in external rotation (figure 8.9*a*). Lift the knee of the internally rotated hip up and move both legs to the other side (figure 8.9*b*), switching the internally rotated hip to now be externally rotated and vice versa. Continue to shift back and forth through the movement, slowly dropping the knees from one side to the other like they are windshield wipers.

> **PRO CUE:** Keep the sit bones on the ground to keep the motion in the hips rather than the spine.

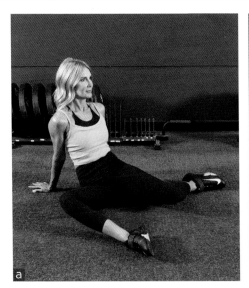 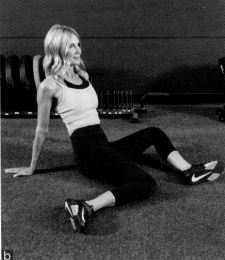

FIGURE 8.9   Windshield wiper 90/90 hip stretch, with *(a)* one hip in internal rotation and the other in external rotation and *(b)* the legs moved to the other side.

HIP FLEXOR MOBILITY WITH ONE-ARM REACH

After sitting all day, and even with walking and running, your hip flexors may tighten. Starting your workout with a hip flexor stretch will get your body in the right position to engage your hips and core. This version adds a twist to increase the stretch even more from the previous phases.

Position

Begin in a half-kneeling position. Bend one leg in front of you, keeping your foot flat on the ground. Your other leg is behind you, your toes tucked under for an active ankle stretch. Hips are square and chest is tall and facing forward.

Movement

With the arm on the same side as the leg you are kneeling on, reach overhead (figure 8.10a). As you reach, exhale and pulse your hips forward, feeling a stretch in the hip flexor of the back leg. During the movement, keep your core engaged, thinking about tucking your belt buckle toward the ceiling. As you are stretching your hip flexors, increase the stretch by reaching up and around toward the back corner of the opposite side, twisting your upper body away from the stretched hip (figure 8.10b). Follow your arm with your eyes to take your entire torso with you. Hold for 30 to 60 seconds, then switch sides.

> **PRO CUE:** Visualize the pelvis being like a bucket full of water; keep the bucket level so water doesn't spill while you perform this movement.

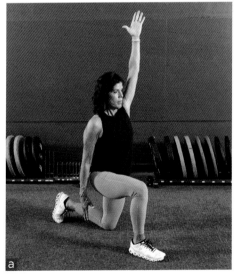 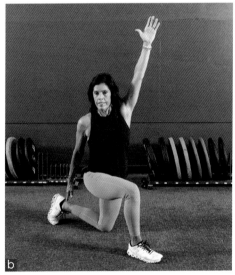

FIGURE 8.10 Hip flexor mobility with one-arm reach, with *(a)* reaching overhead and *(b)* twisting the upper body away from the stretched hip.

TWO-LEG HIP BRIDGE

Time to switch on the posterior chain, firing up the glutes and hamstrings to get ready to work.

Position

Lie on your back with your knees bent and your feet flat on the floor and hip-width apart (figure 8.11a). Arms are externally rotated at your sides.

Movement

With your feet planted, lift your hips off the ground until your knees, hips, and shoulders are in one line (figure 8.11b). Keep the tension out of your neck and shoulders with all the tension in your glutes holding your hips up. Be careful not to hyperextend the lower back. Lower under control and repeat.

PRO CUE: To initiate the movement, "hide" the ribs and then drive the heels into the floor.

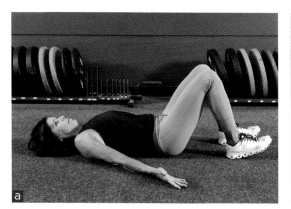 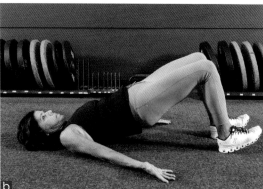

FIGURE 8.11   Two-leg hip bridge, with *(a)* the starting position and *(b)* keeping knees, hips, and shoulders in line.

FROG STRETCH

This exercise will warm up the hips and improve mobility so you can drop into your squats. From the side, it looks like a squat position with motion.

Position

Come into an all-fours position. Place your knees outside of shoulder-width apart then lower onto your forearms (figure 8.12).

Movement

Rock your hips up and down between your feet, as if performing a squat movement while supporting yourself on your forearms. The movement will stretch your inner thighs and externally rotate your hips.

PRO CUE: Use a passive exhale as you move backward and gently use your strength to pull yourself into the stretch.

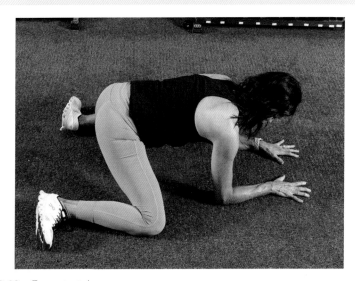

FIGURE 8.12 Frog stretch.

90/90 STRETCH

Continue to work on improving your hip mobility as you stretch, mobilize, and rotate your body over your hips.

Position

Sit on the floor with one leg in front bent at a 90-degree angle and externally rotated and your other leg at a 90-degree angle behind you and internally rotated.

Movement

Keeping your spine in a neutral position, walk your hand over your front knee, then slowly walk your hand toward the front foot (figure 8.13), stopping at five points along the way from the knee to the foot. Switch the legs and repeat on the other side.

> **PRO CUE:** Push the shin of the front leg into the ground. Make your spine long to emphasize motion at the hip rather than the low back.

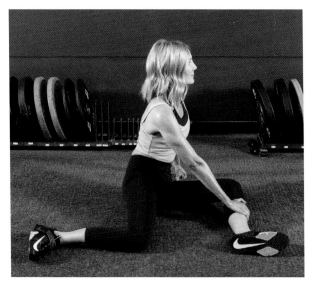

FIGURE 8.13   90/90 stretch.

IN-PLACE SPIDERMAN ON FLOOR OR INCLINE

To get you ready to perform the dynamic Spiderman stretch in later phases of the program, you'll first perform this stationary version to gain mobility and strength.

Position

Begin in a tall plank position with your body held up by your hands and toes (figure 8.14a). Your head, upper back, hips, and feet are in one straight line. In the base phase, it is recommended to start this exercise on an incline, placing your hands on a box or bench, if needed.

Movement

Keeping your body as still as you can, move one foot to outside the hand on that same side of the body, placing your foot flat on the ground while maintaining a neutral spine (figure 8.14b). If you're using a bench or box, place the foot on the ground as close to in line with your hands as possible. The opposite leg remains straight behind you, creating an active stretch of the hip flexor of the back leg. Return that leg to the starting position and repeat with the opposite leg. Alternate for the number of reps.

> **PRO CUE:** Form a straight line from the heel of the back leg to the top of the head. Our colleague Nick Winkelman often says, "From head to heel, straight as steel."

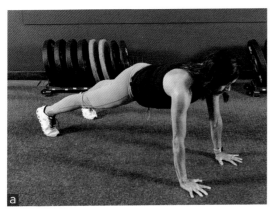
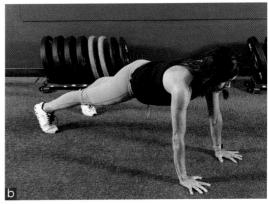

FIGURE 8.14   In-place Spiderman on floor, with *(a)* tall plank position and *(b)* maintaining a neutral spine.

IN-PLACE SPIDERMAN WITH T-REACH

Adding an upper-body reach to the Spiderman drill performed in the base phase helps to increase the stretch, making this a great overall warm-up exercise.

Position

Begin in a plank position with your body held up by your hands and toes (figure 8.15*a*). Your head, upper back, hips, and feet are in one straight line. In the base phase, start this exercise on an incline, placing your hands on a box or bench.

Movement

Keeping your body as still as you can, move one foot to outside the hand on that same side of the body, placing your foot flat on the ground while maintaining a neutral spine. If you're using a bench or box, place the foot on the ground as close to in line with your hands as possible. The opposite leg remains straight behind you, creating an active stretch of the hip flexor of the back leg. Lift the arm on the same side of the front leg to reach for the ceiling, rotating from your upper back to form a T shape with both arms as viewed from the side (figure 8.15*b*). Return to the starting position and repeat with the opposite leg and arm. Alternate for the number of reps.

PRO CUE: Keep the palm of the hand that is reaching up facing toward the front the room. As you look up, you should be able to see your palm. This helps ensure that you are rotating from the upper back.

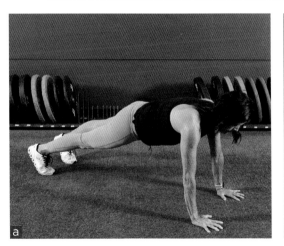 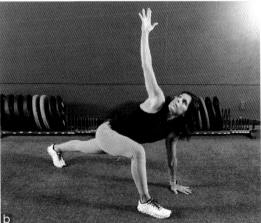

FIGURE 8.15   In-place Spiderman with T-reach, with *(a)* plank position and *(b)* the T shape.

BRIDGE WITH MARCH

This is a progression from the two-leg hip bridge in the base phase warm-up. Now you'll keep the bridge position while you lift one leg and then the other, keeping the core stabilized.

Position

Lie on your back with your knees bent and feet flat on the floor and shoulder-width apart. Arms are externally rotated at your side.

Movement

With your feet planted, lift your hips off the ground until your knees, hips, and shoulders are in one line. Keep the tension out of your neck and shoulders with all the tension in your glutes holding your hips up. Be careful not to hyperextend. Hold that position as you lift one leg off the floor, keeping it bent (figure 8.16), don't let your hips shift. Lower that leg and lift the other leg, alternating back and forth while you keep your hips extended and core as stable as possible.

> **PRO CUE:** When exchanging feet, think of "peeling" the heel off the floor rather than just quickly lifting it. This helps to keep the hips level and square.

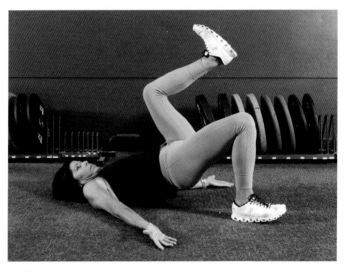

FIGURE 8.16 Bridge with march.

ONE-LEG KNEE HUG HIP BRIDGE

This is a progression from the two-leg hip bridge in the base phase warm-up to performing a one-leg bridge to fire up your posterior chain.

Position

Lie on your back with your knees bent and your feet flat on the floor and shoulder-width apart. Bring one knee into the chest and hug it to your chest with your arms (figure 8.17a).

Movement

Drive through the foot planted on the ground to lift your hips off the ground until your knee, hip, and shoulder are in one line (figure 8.17b). Keep the tension out of your neck and shoulders with all the tension in your glutes, which are holding your hips up. Be careful not to hyperextend. Hold that position and then lower under control. Repeat on that leg for the number of reps and then switch legs.

> **PRO CUE:** You can put a tennis ball just in front of the crease of hip while you hug the knee. This prevents you from cheating the movement by substituting a low-back extension for a hip extension on the other leg.

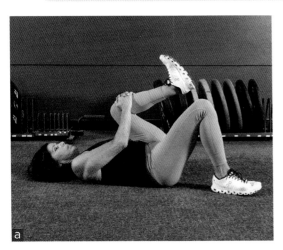 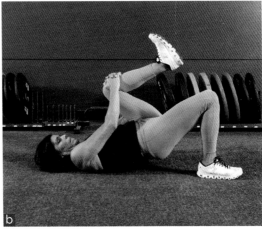

FIGURE 8.17 One-leg knee hug hip bridge, with *(a)* starting position and *(b)* lifting hips until knee, hip, and shoulder are in one line.

THORACIC SPINE MOBILITY

If you're spending lots of time rounded over your desk, leaning toward your computer, or even driving your car, this troublesome posture can be counterbalanced with exercises that wake up your upper-back muscles and stretch the pecs and shoulders as you open up your chest.

SIDE-LYING RIB PULL

This is a self-mobilization exercise that increases the range of motion of the thoracic spine to improve shoulder and hip mobility.

Position

Lie on your side on the floor and flex the top hip to a 90-degree angle. Support the knee of the bent leg with a foam roller or other padded object and support the head on a rolled towel. Keep the opposite leg straight and on the ground (figure 8.18a).

Movement

Reach under your bottom ribs with the top hand. Rotate your top shoulder toward the floor behind you while pulling the ribs in the direction you are rotating (figure 8.18b). Keep the knee in contact with the foam roller or object. Complete the reps on this side, then switch sides.

> **PRO CUE:** Imagine "gluing" your hand to the ribs that you are holding so that the hand does not slide off the ribs while you perform the exercise.

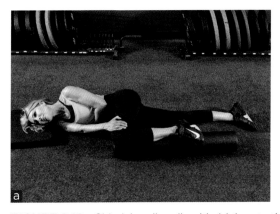 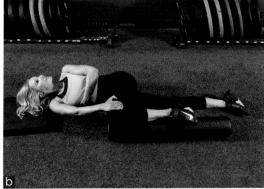

FIGURE 8.18 Side-lying rib pull, with *(a)* the starting position and *(b)* rotating your shoulder toward the floor.

HEEL SIT QUADRUPED THORACIC SPINE EXTERNAL ROTATION

As people age, they may get shorter. This is usually because their posture starts to round over as they lose the strength to hold themselves up. This exercise is the first step to strengthening those upper-back postural muscles while mobilizing your thoracic spine to have tall, proud posture and healthy shoulders. The more you do it, the better you'll get at it.

Position

Begin in a kneeling position on both knees. Sit back on your heels. Round your spine forward, with one forearm on the ground and the palm of that hand face down. Place the other hand on the back of your head with your elbow bent (figure 8.19*a*).

Movement

Push your forearm into the ground. Think about pulling the elbow of the arm on your head back toward the ceiling as you rotate your upper back, allowing your eyes to follow the rotation (figure 8.19*b*). Rotate as far as you can while keeping your opposite arm pressed into the floor and your hips on your heels. Return to the start and complete the repetitions on the same side before switching sides. Each time, try to rotate a little further.

> **PRO CUE:** At your end range of motion, perform a long and slow breath. "Peel" open a bit more on the passive exhale. This lets your body know that it is safe, and you will often gain further range of motion.

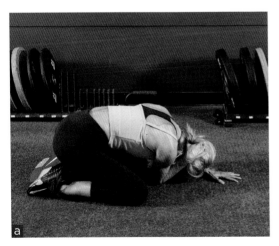 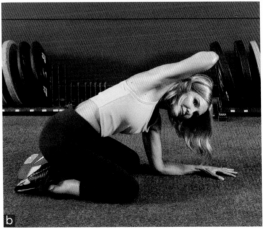

FIGURE 8.19   Heel sit quadruped thoracic spine external rotation, with *(a)* starting position and *(b)* rotating the upper back.

HEEL SIT QUADRUPED ALTERNATING REACH-THROUGH

This exercise will engage your upper-back postural muscles while mobilizing your thoracic spine to have tall proud posture and healthy shoulders.

Position

Begin in a kneeling position on both knees. Sit back on your heels. Place your hands shoulder-width apart on the floor in front of you.

Movement

Lift one arm and thread it through the hole between your other arm and body, reaching to the side (figure 8.20). As you're reaching through, rotate your upper back until the shoulder makes contact with the floor yet maintain the contact between your hips and heels so that the movement is coming from your upper back. Return to the start and repeat on the opposite side. Alternate back and forth for the number of reps. Each time try to rotate a little further.

> **PRO CUE:** Keep the palm up of the arm that is reaching facing the ceiling, and the arm straight.

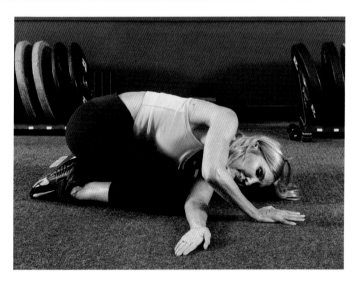

FIGURE 8.20 Heel sit quadruped alternating reach-through.

OPEN HALF-KNEELING POSITION WITH T-REACH

This is one of my favorite warm-up moves, getting your upper back ready along with mobilizing your hips as you connect your upper body to your lower body.

Position

Begin in a half-kneeling position. Turn one leg out to the side, keeping the knee at a 90-degree angle. Bend to place the same hand as your kneeling leg on the floor in line with the knee that is on the ground (figure 8.21*a*).

Movement

Reach your other arm through the hole between the hand touching the floor and your body and then bring the arm up to the ceiling, following it with your eyes to rotate your upper back as you look toward the ceiling. You should form a T shape, with both arms straight, one hand on the floor and one reaching toward the sky (figure 8.21*b*). Repeat on the same side then switch sides.

> **PRO CUE:** Keep the palm of the hand that is reaching up facing toward the front the room. As you look up, you should be able to see the palm. This will help ensure that you are rotating from the upper back.

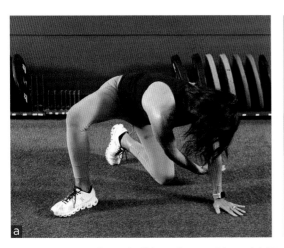
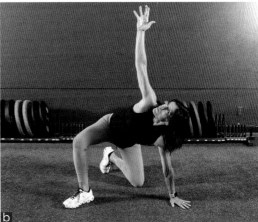

FIGURE 8.21   Open half-kneeling position with T-reach, *(a)* starting position and *(b)* forming a T shape.

ANKLE MOBILITY

Tight ankles will create problems up the chain in your body. Spending time improving mobility at your ankles will improve all of your movements.

OPEN HALF-KNEELING ANKLE MOBILITY

Lacking ankle mobility is one of the number one reasons for compensations leading to injuries up the kinetic chain. Spending some time mobilizing the ankle joint will have you squatting better, lunging better, and overall doing every movement better.

Position

Begin in a half-kneeling position. Turn one leg out to the side, bent at a 90-degree angle.

Movement

Shift your weight forward so that the knee extends past the second toe of that foot while keeping your heel down (figure 8.22). If you feel a stretch in your adductor, your foot is out too far; bring the foot closer to you and work on easing the knee forward to improve ankle mobility. Pulse out and hold for 3 seconds each repetition. Repeat on the other side.

> **PRO CUE:** Imagine the heel of the shoe is superglued or cemented to the ground during the movement. Lifting the heel is cheating the movement.

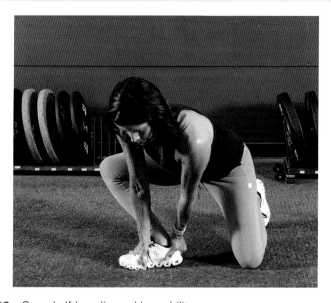

FIGURE 8.22   Open half-kneeling ankle mobility.

FLOOR PIKE ALTERNATING ANKLE MOBILITY

This is one of my favorite warm-up exercises because it improves ankle mobility and warms up your hamstrings, upper back, and shoulders while engaging your core to get ready for your workout. I always feel realigned after this one.

Position

Begin in a plank position with your body held up by your hands and toes (figure 8.23*a*). Your head, upper back, hips, and feet are in one straight line.

Movement

Lift your hips as you push the heel of one leg toward the floor, increasing the range of motion at the ankle joint while your head drops between your arms. Bend the other leg, putting all your weight on the leg you are actively stretching (figure 8.23*b*). That leg stays straight; feel a stretch in your hamstrings right into the calf and ankle. Switch and bend the opposite leg, straightening and stretching the ankle, calf, and hamstring. Then rock back down to a plank position to complete one repetition. Repeat for the number of desired repetitions.

> **PRO CUE:** Imagine that both feet are on their own narrow balance beams during this movement. They must stay pointed straight ahead and should not turn outward.

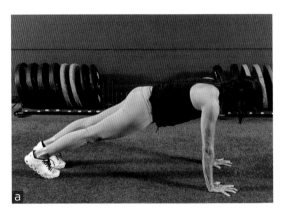
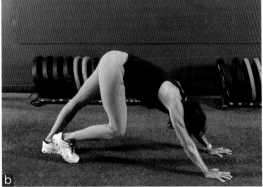

FIGURE 8.23   Floor pike alternating ankle mobility, with *(a)* plank position and *(b)* putting all your weight on the leg you are actively stretching.

WALL ANKLE MOBILITY DRILL

This drill gives you another option to increase your ankle mobility. The ankle is such a crucial joint to have full mobility with, because if you don't have full mobility, you'll compensate up the chain, causing injury.

Position

Stand facing a wall with your hands on the wall. Place your feet about 1 to 2 inches from the wall, and then step one foot back 2 to 3 more inches.

Movement

Bend the knee of the back leg over the toes, reaching the knee toward the wall while keeping the heel down and mobilizing the ankle (figure 8.24). If you cannot touch your knee to the wall without raising your heel, move your foot a bit closer so you are just grazing the wall. As you improve your ankle mobility, you'll be able to start farther from the wall. Pulse the knee over the toes each time, trying to get a little closer to the wall. Repeat for the desired number of repetitions, then switch to the other side.

> **PRO CUE:** Imagine that the heel of the shoe is superglued or cemented to the ground during the movement. Lifting the heel is cheating the movement.

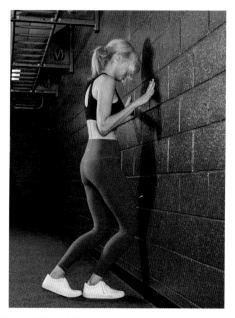

FIGURE 8.24   Wall ankle mobility drill.

COMBINATION OF MOVEMENTS

Performing a combination of movements as part of your warm-up is a great way to integrate everything together into movement while raising your core temperature and increasing your heart rate.

WORLD'S GREATEST STRETCH: LUNGE WITH HAMSTRING STRETCH AND T-REACH

This is an all-in-one move combining three different mobility drills. It was named the World's Greatest Stretch by renowned strength coach Mark Verstegen of Exos.

Position

Stand with your feet hip-width apart.

Movement

Step forward into a lunge with one leg while bending down until your hands are on the ground, one on each side of the front leg. Keep the back leg straight, creating a hip flexor stretch of the back hip (figure 8.25*a*). In that position, reach the same arm as the front leg up to the ceiling, rotating your upper body to open your hips and upper back (figure 8.25*b*). Return your hand to the floor and then rock your hips back, straightening your front leg as much as you can while keeping your hands on the floor, pulling your front toe off the ground to feel a stretch in the front calf all the way up that back leg (figure 8.25*c*). Return to standing and repeat on the other side.

> **PRO CUE:** Think of slightly lifting your back pockets to the ceiling during the hamstring stretch portion of the movement. The pro cues from the Spiderman variations apply to the other portions of this movement as well.

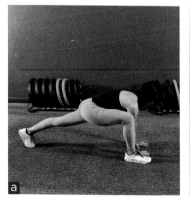 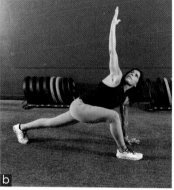 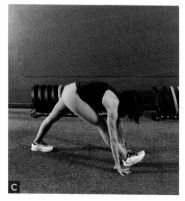

FIGURE 8.25 World's greatest stretch: lunge with hamstring stretch and T-reach, with *(a)* stepping forward into the lunge, *(b)* opening your hips and upper back, and *(c)* feeling the stretch in the calf.

OPEN HALF-KNEELING WINDMILL

From the open half-kneeling with T-reach move you learned earlier in the chapter, you'll easily transition to this "feels so good" move to get some dynamic hip mobility and upper-back rotation happening before you try your first Turkish get-up (coming up next).

Position

Begin in a half-kneeling position. Turn one leg out to the side, keeping the knee at a 90-degree angle.

Movement

Bend to place the same hand as the knee on the ground on the floor in front of and in line with the knee on the ground while you reach the opposite arm up to the ceiling so that your arms form a straight line from the ground toward the ceiling (figure 8.26a). You'll feel the stretch in the outside of your hip as you think about hinging it behind you. Lift the hand on the ground as you bring your upper body back to an upright position with tall posture, keeping one arm straight overhead and the other arm hanging down (figure 8.26b). Return that same hand to the ground as you rotate your upper back to reach the other arm for the ceiling, again hinging at the hip and forming that straight line (figure 8.26c). If this feels too easy, take the arm on the floor all the way down to the forearm to increase the stretch at the hip and upper back. Repeat for the number of reps and then switch sides.

> **PRO CUE:** Imagine you are holding a 100-pound kettlebell in the top hand. This will help you keep that arm vertical while you perform the windmill.

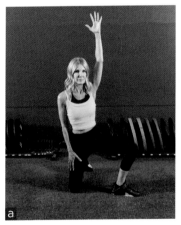 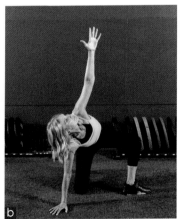 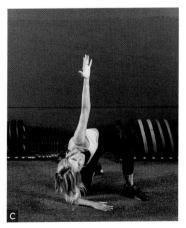

FIGURE 8.26 Open half-kneeling windmill with *(a)* the arms forming a straight line from ground to ceiling, *(b)* one arm is straight overhead and one arm is down, and *(c)* hinging at the hip and forming a straight line.

TURKISH GET-UP

If there's a most-bang-for-your-buck exercise, this is it. Talk about working the full body. You'll be tying together all the movements you've been practicing. Take your time with this one because each step of this exercise accomplishes something. As you get stronger, you'll be able to add load by holding a kettlebell. I highly recommend you work with a coach to help you learn proper form on this one because there is a lot going on.

Position

Lie on your back on the ground. Bend one knee so your foot is flat on the floor, with the arm on the same side as the bent leg reaching straight up toward the ceiling (figure 8.27a).

Movement

Step 1: Keep the raised arm vertical as you press into the foot that is flat on the ground. Roll diagonally to the forearm of the other arm (figure 8.27b). Keep your chest up and your shoulders down, away from your ears.

Step 2: Press up from your forearm to place your weight on your hand with your arm straight; the raised arm continues to reach straight up to the ceiling as you sit on the hip of your straight leg (figure 8.27c).

Step 3: Sweep your straight leg through to an open half-kneeling position behind you, lifting your hips off the ground while still reaching the raised arm to the ceiling and keeping your weight on the forearm (figure 8.27d). You'll finish this step in an open half-kneeling position with the same hand as the foot that is on the ground supporting you and the raised arm reaching toward the ceiling.

Step 4: Bring your body upright so you are in an open half-kneeling position, with your arm still reaching overhead and your other arm now hanging (figure 8.27e). Lift the chest with a tall, proud posture. Pivot the rear leg in a move called a "windshield wiper" and square off to a half-kneeling position. At this point you can reverse the movement back to the floor or continue to the next step.

Step 5: Drive through the front foot to stand all the way up (figure 8.27f). Reverse each step to lower yourself back to the lying position. Repeat for the number of reps on each side.

PRO CUE: Think of the first part of the get-up as a full-body diagonal roll rather than a traditional sit-up.

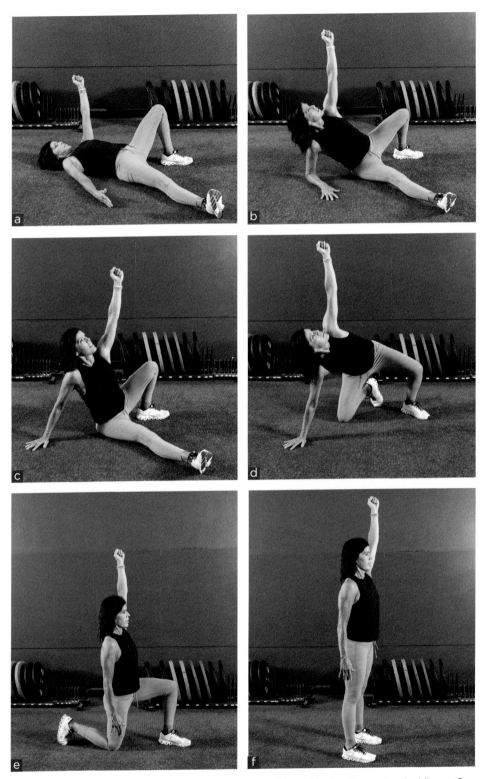

FIGURE 8.27 Turkish get-up with *(a)* starting position, *(b)* step 1, *(c)* step 2, *(d)* step 3, *(e)* step 4, and *(f)* step 5.

PATTERNING (HIP HINGE)

Bending at the hip is one of the most important movements to include in your workout to strengthen your posterior chain. It's important to warm up the movement before you load to improve your form and use the right muscles.

BODYWEIGHT PRISONER RDL

Learn to do a proper hip hinge with this warm-up move. Romanian deadlifts can be difficult to learn; this version with only your body weight will help you nail Romanian deadlifts in the training program.

Position

Stand tall, your feet just outside of shoulder-width apart, your hands on the back of your head, and your elbows out (figure 8.28*a*).

Movement

Shifting your weight back, hinge forward at the hips (figure 8.28*b*). Imagine reaching your hips toward a wall behind you. Keep your chest up and your spine long as your upper body hinges forward without any rounding. Reverse the movement to return to standing.

> **PRO CUE:** Imagine you are standing with your hips in the center of a compass, facing north. Visualize pushing your back pockets straight back to south.

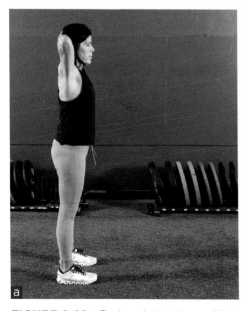 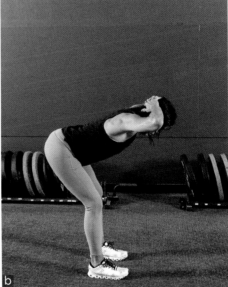

FIGURE 8.28 Bodyweight prisoner RDL.

BODYWEIGHT STAGGERED-STANCE RDL

This drill takes the hip-hinge movement you learned in phase one, the bodyweight prisoner RDL, and brings you to a staggered-stance. This will eventually lead to balancing on a single leg.

Position

Stand tall, with your feet hip-width apart, your hands on the back of your head, and your elbows out. Slide one foot back so that the toes of that foot are in line with the heel of the other foot (figure 8.29*a*), putting most of your weight on the foot in front.

Movement

Shifting your weight back, hinge forward at the hips. Imagine reaching your hips toward a wall behind you (figure 8.29*b*). Keep your chest up and your spine long as your upper body hinges forward without any rounding at the spine. Your weight is unevenly distributed, with more weight on your front leg while the back leg provides support. Reverse the movement to return to standing.

> **PRO CUE:** Imagine you are wearing a ski boot on the front leg. Most of your weight will be on this leg. A common error is to shift your weight onto the back leg while pushing the hips back.

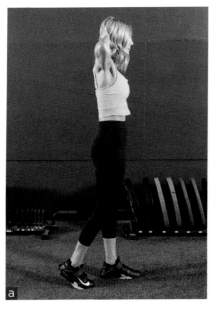 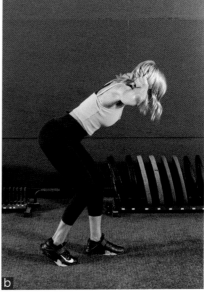

FIGURE 8.29   Bodyweight staggered-stance RDL, with *(a)* starting position and *(b)* reaching your hips back while hinging forward.

BODYWEIGHT ONE-LEG RDL

This warm-up exercise switches on your stabilizer muscles and nervous system as you balance while providing active hamstring mobility.

Position

Stand tall with your feet hip-width apart (figure 8.30*a*).

Movement

Shift your weight to one leg, keeping a slight bend in the knee, and push the hips back as you reach the opposite arm diagonally across your body toward the ground. The raised leg lifts behind you as you balance on your standing leg (figure 8.30*b*), engaging your stabilizers and actively stretching the hamstring. The reach in this movement helps to keep the hips squared to the ground. Return to the start position and repeat on the other side.

> **PRO CUE:** Your standing (nonmoving or nonworking leg) must have a slight bend. This is essential to allow a posterior weight shift. Visualize leaving a low footprint on the wall behind you as you hinge forward.

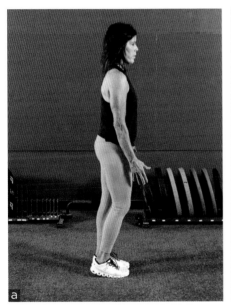 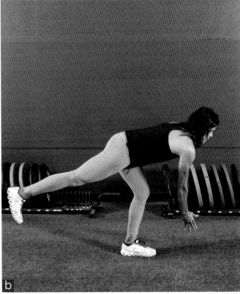

FIGURE 8.30 Bodyweight one-leg RDL, with *(a)* starting position and *(b)* balancing on your standing leg.

| **Variation:** | Bodyweight One-Leg Tempo RDL |

Balance is one of the key things to train as we age, with falling being the biggest risk to ending up in the hospital. This exercise will train your balance along with waking up your posterior chain, working your butt and hamstrings to keep you strong.

Stand with your feet shoulder-width apart. Shift your weight to balance on one leg. Chest is up as you stand with tall posture. Shift your weight to your standing leg as you push the hips back, lifting the free leg and sending your hips behind you as your torso bends forward. Maintain a neutral spine; avoid any rounding. If you can't touch your hand to the floor without rounding your back, place an object such as a cone to reach to. Slowly return to the starting position and repeat on the same leg for the number of reps before switching legs.

Your standing (nonmoving or nonworking leg) must have a slight bend. This is essential to allow a posterior weight shift to occur. Visualize leaving a low footprint on the wall behind you as you lower yourself.

PATTERNING (ASYMMETRICAL SQUAT)

Working on some of the movement patterns that will show up in your workout, including the squat movement, with this asymmetrical squat will get you prepared for what's to come.

TALL KNEEL TO HALF KNEEL

If you lack balance and stability when you stand on one leg, these half-kneeling and tall-kneeling positions will help! By transitioning between the two in this move while training the core to remain stable, you'll notice fast results. We use them both a lot at Results Fitness and throughout this program. As part of the base phase warm-up, you will practice these positions. The half-kneeling position with hip flexion and extension around a strong stable core resembles so many of the advanced progressions, such as lunges. From a half-kneeling position, when you bring your front foot toward the midline of your body, you'll quickly notice any asymmetries or discrepancies as you may find that you lose your balance or have to kick your hip out to maintain balance. This exercise builds the stability you need in the bottom of a lunge or split squat position.

Position

Start in a tall-kneeling position on both knees (figure 8.31a).

Movement

Keeping your core as stable as possible with very little movement, bring one leg through to the half-kneeling position in front of you (figure 8.31b). Return to the starting tall-kneeling position and repeat with the opposite leg, alternating back and forth into the half-kneeling position, paying attention each time to keeping the connection between your hips, torso, and shoulders.

PRO CUE: Stay tall and vertical while switching legs. Imagine someone is holding on to your hair tightly while you are performing this movement. The goal is to keep any of your hair from being pulled out!

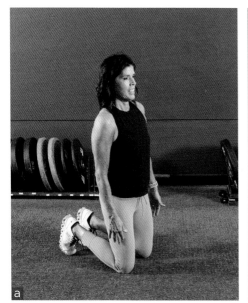 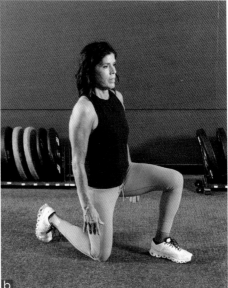

FIGURE 8.31   Tall kneel to half kneel, with *(a)* starting position and *(b)* bringing one leg to half-kneeling position.

SUSPENSION TRAINER STATIONARY SPLIT SQUAT

Since you've been improving your balance and flexibility, you're ready to include split squats, a staple exercise that can progress into dynamic lunges and reverse lunges. Use a suspension trainer to support some of your body weight.

Position

Start in a half-kneeling position, bringing one leg forward. The front knee and hip are at a 90-degree angle. The back leg will also be at 90 degrees on the floor (figure 8.32*a*).

Movement

Holding the suspension trainer handles, brace the core and dig the back toe into the ground as you stand up to the top of a split squat position (figure 8.32*b*). Use the suspension trainer as much or as little as needed. Lower until your knee is just off the ground and repeat on the same leg before switching legs.

> **PRO CUE:** Keep your hips level and square front to back and side to side while performing this movement. It is helpful to think of this drill as a "moving" half-kneeling plank where you move mostly up and down and not forward and backward.

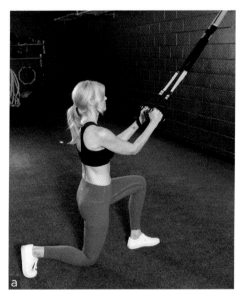 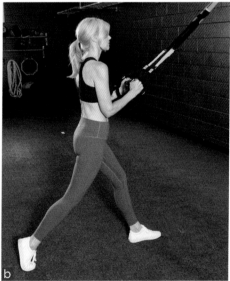

FIGURE 8.32   Suspension trainer stationary split squat, with *(a)* starting position and *(b)* standing up to the top of a split squat.

REVERSE LUNGE WITH ROTATION

After getting dynamic with the lunge pattern, practicing your split squats and getting stronger, you're now ready to hit a reverse lunge as part of your warm-up. This exercise actively stretches the hip flexors while firing up the lower body. Adding the rotation even wakes up the upper back.

Position

Stand with your feet hip-width apart, your hands behind your head, and your elbows bent (figure 8.33a). Keep a tall posture and proud chest with your shoulders down and back.

Movement

Shift your weight to one side as you step the other leg behind you and lower into a lunge. Do not narrow your stance, or it will make it more difficult to balance. Lower until the back knee almost touches the floor, and rotate your upper body toward the back leg (figure 8.33b). Brace your abs to keep the pelvis stable as you lunge. Push through the front foot to return to the start position. Alternate sides for the number of reps.

PRO CUE: Keep the forward leg frozen, as if it's in cement, while rotating.

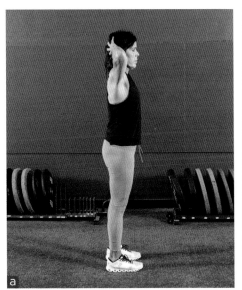 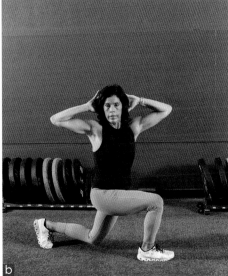

FIGURE 8.33   Reverse lunge with rotation, with *(a)* starting position and *(b)* rotating the upper body toward the back leg.

LATERAL SQUAT

It's important to warm up your adductors so that you can use your hips properly during your workout. The lateral squat does this.

Position

Stand with your feet well outside of shoulder-width apart.

Movement

Bend one leg as you send your hips back, keeping the opposite leg straight, shifting your body to the side of the bent leg as you squat down (figure 8.34). Go as deep as you can, bending the working leg as low as you can while keeping your heel on the floor. Return to the start by straightening the leg, and repeat on the same side for the number of reps before switching sides.

> **PRO CUE:** Allow your torso to lean forward naturally during this movement. The back should be stable and straight but not vertical. You must lean forward to counterbalance yourself. Keep the knee joint stacked over the ankle joint.

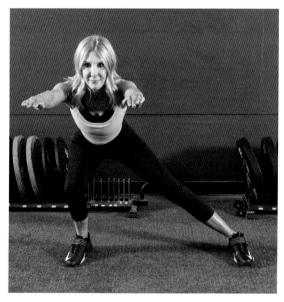

FIGURE 8.34   Lateral squat.

ALTERNATING LATERAL SQUAT

This exercise takes the lateral squat and shifts it back and forth, alternating sides, making it a more dynamic movement.

Position

Stand with your feet outside of shoulder-width apart.

Movement

Bend one leg to the side, sending your hips back, keeping the opposite leg straight, and shifting your body to the side of the bent leg as you squat down. Go as deep as you can, bending the working leg. Go only as low as you can while keeping your heel on the floor. Drive off that leg to bring it back to the starting position and shift to the opposite side, keeping your feet planted as you alternate from one side to the other.

> **PRO CUE:** Allow your torso to lean forward naturally during this movement. Your back should be stable and straight but not vertical. You must lean forward to counterbalance yourself. Keep the knee joint stacked over the ankle joint.

LOW LATERAL SQUAT

This is one more exercise to warm up your adductors and prepare your hips for your workout. This move takes the lateral squat you've progressed from stationary to dynamic to keep you in the deep squat position the entire time as you shift back and forth. If you're not ready for this, stick with the alternating lateral squat.

Position

Stand tall with your feet outside of shoulder-width apart.

Movement

Bend one leg to the side, sending your hips back. Keep the opposite leg straight as you shift your body to the side of the bent leg and squat. Go as deep as you can, bending the working leg, but go only as low as you can while keeping your heel down. To perform this version, you'll need to be able to squat low with your heel down because you'll be staying in that position without coming back up. You can rotate the heel of the opposite foot off the ground to get more range. Instead of driving off the working leg to return to the start position, you'll stay low and slowly shift your weight to the middle and then to the opposite side so you're staying in the full squat position the entire time, shifting from one side to the other (figure 8.35). Repeat back and forth, staying in the full squat position with your heel down on the working leg and the opposite leg straight with the heel rotated up to increase range of motion.

> **PRO CUE:** Allow your torso to lean forward naturally during this movement. The back should be stable and straight but not vertical. You must lean forward to counterbalance yourself. Keep the knee joint stacked over the ankle joint.

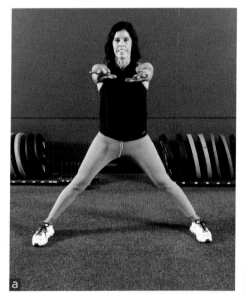 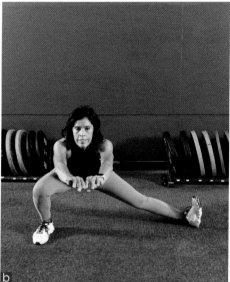

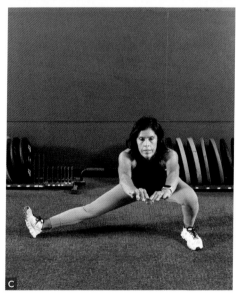

FIGURE 8.35 Low lateral squat.

PATTERNING (SYMMETRICAL SQUAT)

Working on the movement patterns you'll be doing in your workout, including the symmetrical squat, will get your body ready for what's to come.

SUSPENSION TRAINER SQUAT PRYING

Using a suspension trainer such as a TRX to hold your body weight while performing a lunge or squat is a very good way to make those exercises easier and train the movement properly as you're building strength.

Position

Stand in front of a suspension trainer with your feet just outside of shoulder-width apart. Grab the handles of the suspension trainer.

Movement

Lower yourself into a full squat with your hips between your legs, your heels down, and your chest up as you support some of your body weight with the suspension trainer (figure 8.36). Stay in the squat position and rock back and forth, really warming up the squat position; this is also known as *prying*. Return to the standing position and repeat.

> **PRO CUE:** Prying is simply making small motions to create space in the joints. Keep the knees tracking the toes while making prying motions in the squat.

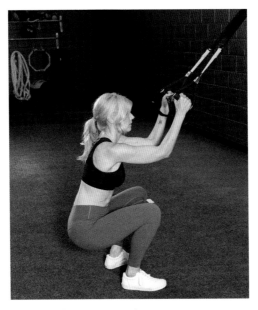

FIGURE 8.36 Suspension trainer squat prying.

TOE TOUCH TO FROG SQUAT

Squatting is one of our most primal movements. Babies demonstrate a perfect mobile squat because that is how they stand up: from a crawl to a squat to standing up. Keeping the ability to squat is important for anti-aging. Our ability to get off the floor has a direct correlation to the length and quality of our lives. This movement gets your squat movement ready to go.

Position

Stand tall with your feet shoulder-width apart and slightly turned out.

Movement

Bend over and grab your toes, keeping your legs straight (figure 8.37a). Bend your knees as you drop your hips between your legs, lifting your chest as if showing the logo on your T-shirt at the bottom of the squat (figure 8.37b). Keep your heels on the ground as you squat. Your arms should be inside your knees, holding the toes. As you hold the toes, straighten the legs to lift the hips, dropping the head down back to the toe touch position. Repeat.

> **PRO CUE:** At the bottom of the squat, imagine that you have laser beams coming out of your eyes; you want those laser beams to project straight ahead to the wall in front of you.

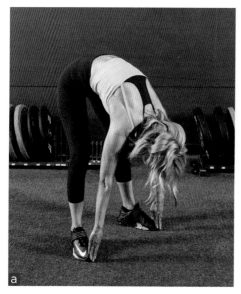 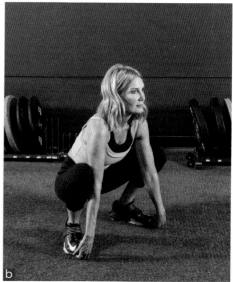

FIGURE 8.37 Toe touch to frog squat, with *(a)* keeping your legs straight and *(b)* lifting your chest.

TOE TOUCH TO BODYWEIGHT SQUAT

This movement builds on the toe touch to frog squat, adding a standing position to strengthen and warm up the muscles used in the squat movement.

Position

Stand tall with your feet shoulder-width apart and your feet slightly turned out.

Movement

Bend over and grab your toes, keeping your legs straight (figure 8.38a). Drop your hips between your legs, lifting your chest as if to show the logo on your T-shirt at the bottom of the squat (figure 8.38b). Keep your heels on the ground as you squat. Your arms should be inside your knees, holding the toes. Let go of the toes and hold your arms straight out in front of you as you get ready to stand (figure 8.38c). Drive through your feet as you stand with your arms straight out in front of you (figure 8.38d). Repeat from the start for the number of reps.

> **PRO CUE:** Once you reach your arms out in front of you at the bottom of the squat, pause for a beat to demonstrate that you own that position on each and every rep.

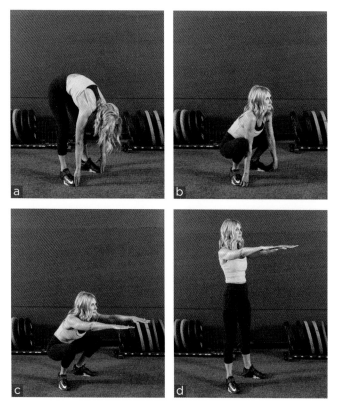

FIGURE 8.38   Toe touch to bodyweight squat, with *(a)* keeping your legs straight *(b)* lifting your chest, *(c)* getting ready to stand, and *(d)* standing up.

TOE TOUCH TO SQUAT WITH OVERHEAD REACH

As your training progresses through the phases of the Age Strong program, you will perform an overhead squat as part of your warm-up.

Position

Stand tall with your feet shoulder-width apart and slightly turned out, and your arms overhead.

Movement

Bend over and grab your toes, keeping your legs straight (figure 8.39*a*). Drop your hips between your legs, lifting your chest as if to show the logo on your T-shirt at the bottom of the squat (figure 8.39*b*). Keep your heels down on the ground as you squat. Your arms should be inside your knees, holding the toes. Let go of the toes and lift your arms overhead while still in the squat position as you get ready to stand (figure 8.39*c*). Drive through your feet as you stand with your arms overhead (figure 8.39*d*), returning to the start position. Repeat for the desired number of reps.

> **PRO CUE:** Once you lift your arms at the bottom of the squat, pause for a beat to demonstrate that you own that position on each and every rep.

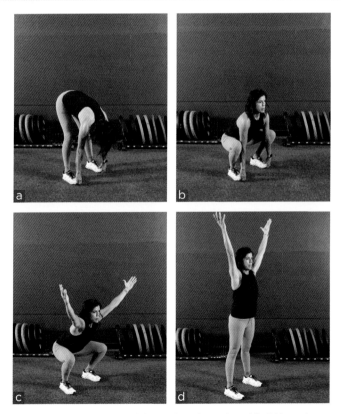

FIGURE 8.39 Toe touch to squat with overhead reach, with *(a)* keeping your legs straight, *(b)* lifting your chest, *(c)* getting ready to stand, and *(d)* standing.

MOVEMENT SKILLS

It's time to start moving faster and finish off your warm-up with some movement skills to be ready as you head into your workout.

HIGH-KNEE MARCH IN PLACE

Time to start moving, elevating the heart rate and getting the blood flowing with a march.

Position

Stand tall, your feet shoulder-width apart.

Movement

Lift one knee as you drive the opposite arm up (figure 8.40), then stamp the foot down. Continue to switch legs and arms to alternate marching.

> **PRO CUE:** Stay tall; if you are 5 feet 5 inches, try to be 5 feet 6 inches while marching.

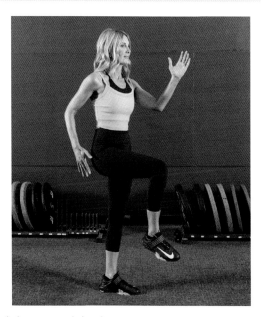

FIGURE 8.40   High-knee march in place.

LATERAL SHUFFLE

After practicing your base position with your knees bent outside of shoulder-width while taking an athletic stance, let's take the movement lateral. This shuffle requires you to push off the working leg as you improve your dynamic lateral movement.

Position

Stand in an athletic position with your feet outside shoulder-width, your knees bent as if you're ready to jump, your hips back, and your chest up (figure 8.41a).

Movement

Move to the left as you drive off the right leg, reaching with the left leg (figure 8.41b). Land with your feet the same distance apart as in the start position. Continue to shuffle in the same direction for the number of reps, then repeat on the other side as you move in the opposite direction.

> **PRO CUE:** Make sure that this is a push into the floor with the trailing leg; it should not be a step and pull with the front leg.

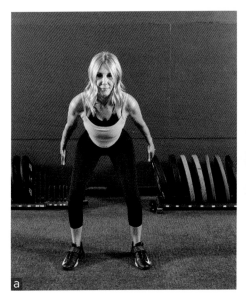 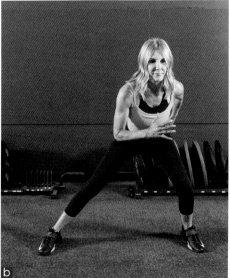

FIGURE 8.41 Lateral shuffle, with *(a)* starting position and *(b)* moving to the left.

LINEAR SKIP

Skippidee doo-da! Ready to feel like a kid again? When was the last time you skipped? Skipping will complement your warm-up with movement integration and linear speed to fire up the nervous system.

Position

Stand tall with your feet shoulder-width apart.

Movement

Similar to the marching exercise, swing one leg and the opposite arm up. Add a hop off each foot as you move forward (figure 8.42), popping yourself off the ground with power.

PRO CUE: Skip in place before trying to do it moving.

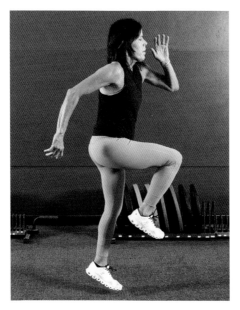

FIGURE 8.42   Linear skip.

LATERAL SKIP

This lateral dynamic movement will keep you agile and ready for your workout.

Position

Stand tall with your feet shoulder-width apart and ready to skip.

Movement

Start with a lateral marching movement, lifting the knee on the side of the direction you'll be moving while pumping the opposite arm up. As you step down with the outside leg, raise the other knee and other arm, moving sideways in a march. Add a hop and you'll find yourself doing a lateral skip (figure 8.43). Think about powering through each step to drive yourself into the air. Repeat for the number of reps in one direction, and then switch direction.

> **PRO CUE:** Push off the trailing leg. It is very helpful to repeat "push" to yourself while you learn this movement.

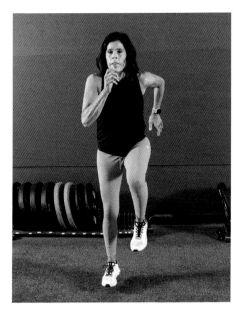

FIGURE 8.43   Lateral skip.

NEURAL ACTIVATION

Ready to get your nervous system firing on all cylinders to head into your workout ready to go? These next exercises will do just that.

DROP TO BASE

Base is the athletic stance we all know from most sports as the stable position an athlete takes with their feet wide, their hips low, and their chest up, ready to move.

Position

Stand with your feet shoulder-width apart.

Movement

Reach both arms overhead and fully extend your body, coming up onto your toes (figure 8.44*a*). Quickly drop to the base athletic position with your feet wide, your hips in a squat, and your chest up (figure 8.44*b*). Shake it out and return to the starting position. Repeat for the desired number of repetitions.

> **PRO CUE:** Imagine that you are standing on a trap door that suddenly opens and closes.

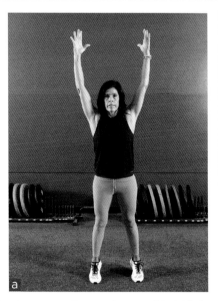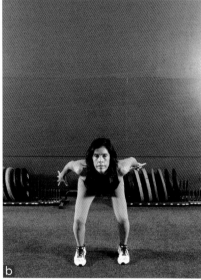

FIGURE 8.44 Drop to base, with *(a)* fully extending your body and *(b)* dropping to the base athletic position.

2 FEET OUT AND IN RUNNING IN PLACE

After performing drop to base for the number of reps, you'll be ready to stay in the base position and move those feet! Let's get that nervous system firing up!

Position

Stand in the base athletic position with your feet wide, your hips lowered into a partial squat, and your chest up.

Movement

Staying in the base position, run as fast as possible as you shuffle the feet with quick movements, 2 feet out and 2 feet in (figure 8.45).

PRO CUE: Think "slow arms and fast feet." The feet will pop back and forth, 2 feet out and 2 feet in.

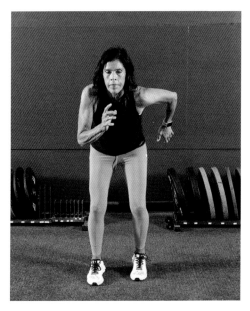

FIGURE 8.45 2 feet out and in running in place.

SPRINT IN PLACE

Let's get your body warm, your heart rate up, and your nervous system knowing it's go time.

Position

Stand tall with the arms bent at the elbows.

Movement

Run in place with quick feet, your arms working in opposition (figure 8.46).

PRO CUE: Drive the knees as if breaking glass above them at the middle of your thigh.

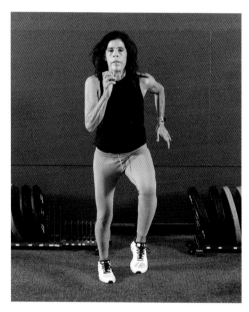

FIGURE 8.46   Sprint in place.

CONCLUSION

A dynamic warm-up prepares your body for the work to come by gradually increasing the range of motion, activating muscles, and shadowing body movements to be loaded in the workout. Don't try to save time by skipping your warm-up. A strong workout is built on a proper warm-up.

CHAPTER 9

CORE

This chapter is full of some of the best core stabilization and strengthening exercises. When done properly, they will engage and strengthen the muscles of the core, where all movement comes from. Over time, due to sitting, surgeries, childbirth, and various other life circumstances, women can lose core strength and the ability to hold a stabilized position, often leading to injuries. These exercises are early in each program because core stabilization and strength are important priorities.

FRONT PLANK

You won't see sit-ups in this program because the most effective core exercises are stabilization exercises. This means you'll be working to keep your trunk as still as possible while performing the movement.

Position

Begin on the floor with your body weight supported on your forearms and toes (figure 9.1). Your palms are down to grip the floor, and your head, shoulders, upper back, and hips are in alignment. Your elbows are positioned directly under your shoulders.

Movement

You won't actually move during this exercise, but you will be working. We often tell our clients that it doesn't look like a lot is happening on the outside, but there is a lot happening on the inside of a properly performed plank! Think about pulling your elbows toward your toes as you brace your core. If you look down and see your abdomen pooching toward the floor like a tent, think about bringing the ribs down toward the hips to engage the deep muscles of your abdominals without lifting your hips. Return your head to the aligned position for the duration of the exercise. Hold for 30 seconds to start, working up to 60 seconds as you progress.

PRO CUE: Visualize your body being stiff, like a surfboard that someone could stand on.

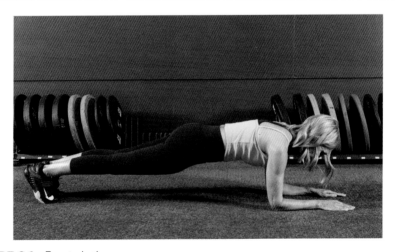

FIGURE 9.1   Front plank.

Variation: Elevated Front Plank

If you find it difficult to perform a front plank on the floor, place your elbows on a bench or step. The elevation will make the plank easier. Once you've improved your strength, you can lower to the floor.

ALTERNATING ONE-LEG FRONT PLANK

This is a progression from the plank, adding in a leg extension while stabilizing the trunk. With each progression of the plank, remember the fundamentals you learned and focus on stabilizing your body.

Position

Begin on the floor with your body weight supported by your forearms and toes. Your palms are down to grip the floor. Your elbows are positioned directly under your shoulders.

Movement

Shift your weight (without perceptible movement) while stabilizing your body to lift one foot off the floor, extending from the hip only as high as you can go without losing alignment (figure 9.2). Think of the front of your hip bones facing the floor at all times. Pause and return to the start position, then repeat with the other leg. Do your best to not move your trunk or hips while performing this exercise.

> PRO CUE: Keep the distance between the ribs and hips the same while moving the legs; it should not increase so that the ribcage won't flailing open, causing you to lose your core stability.

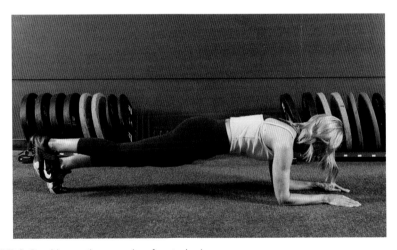

FIGURE 9.2   Alternating one-leg front plank.

GLUTE BRIDGE WITH CABLE CORE ACTIVATION

Position

Lie on your back with your head close to a dual-cable machine, your feet away from the machine, and both handles lowered to the ground at shoulder-width above your head. Both legs are bent with your feet flat on the floor. Grab the handles to pull the load off the weight stack and straighten your arms to the ceiling, activating the core.

Movement

While holding the weight with your arms and engaging your core, lift your hips off the floor (figure 9.3) for the prescribed number of reps.

> **PRO CUE:** Keep your shoulders away from your ears, putting the tension in your core instead of your traps.

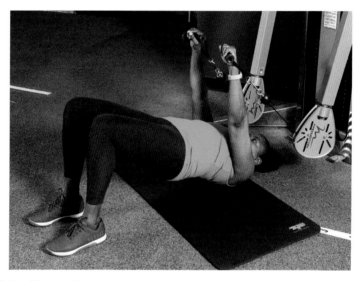

FIGURE 9.3 Glute bridge with cable core activation.

ALTERNATING ARM REACH FRONT PLANK

This is a progression from the plank, adding in an arm reach while stabilizing the trunk. With each progression of the plank, remember the fundamentals and focus on stabilizing your body.

Position

Begin on the floor with your body weight supported by your forearms and toes. Your palms are down to grip the floor, and your elbows are positioned directly under your shoulders.

Movement

Shift your weight while stabilizing your body as you lift one hand off the floor, extending your arm until it's in line with your ear (figure 9.4). Think of the front of your hip bones facing the floor at all times. Pause and then return to the start position. Repeat with the other arm. Do your best to not move your trunk while performing this exercise.

> **PRO CUE:** Imagine you are balancing a cup full of coffee on your lower back while you shift your weight and reach with your arm.

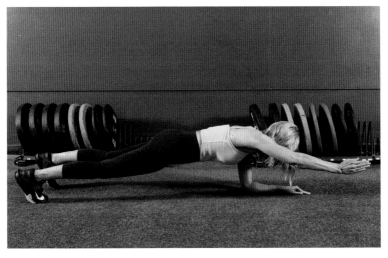

FIGURE 9.4   Alternating arm reach front plank.

SANDBAG ISO KNEELING SIDE PLANK

Before moving into a side plank variation with your legs straight, you'll first work on the side plank variation with bent knees. Using a sandbag (which is optional) to create extra tension, you'll be sure to engage the right muscles to stabilize your body in this side position.

Position

Place a light sandbag on the floor (optional). Lie on your side with the sandbag in front of you, your knees bent and your weight supported by your hip, forearm, and the side of your leg. Your elbow should be stacked directly under your shoulder, with your knees stacked on top of each other (figure 9.5a).

Movement

Engage your core and lift your hips off the ground so that your weight is only supported by your forearm and lower leg, forming a straight line from your head, hips, and knees. As you lift your hips, start to pick up the sandbag (without actually fully picking it up) with your top arm while using the muscles in your back to brace yourself from being pulled forward (figure 9.5b). Hold this position for 30 seconds, working up to 60 seconds. Repeat on the other side.

> **PRO CUE:** Imagine that your body is between two panes of glass to keep your body in a straight line as you hold the position.

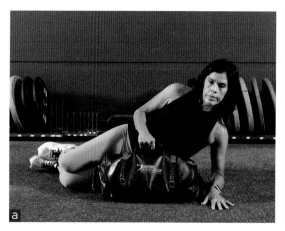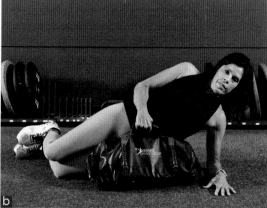

FIGURE 9.5   Sandbag iso kneeling side plank.

SIDE PLANK

This is a progression from the kneeling plank. You'll have only one arm and one foot in contact with the ground, creating less stability and thus making the exercise more challenging. You'll use your core muscles to stabilize your body in this side position.

Position

Lie on your side with your weight supported by your hip, forearm, and the side of your bottom leg. Your elbow should be stacked directly under your shoulder, your legs extended with your feet stacked on top of each other or staggered for more stability. Your top arm can either rest along your side or extend toward the ceiling for balance.

Movement

Engage your core and lift your hips off the ground so that your weight is supported only by your forearm and foot, forming a straight line from your head, hips, and feet (figure 9.6). Hold this position for 30 seconds, working up to 60 seconds. Repeat on the other side.

> **PRO CUE:** Remember, the head and neck are a part of the spine. Keep them lined up with the spine for ideal alignment.

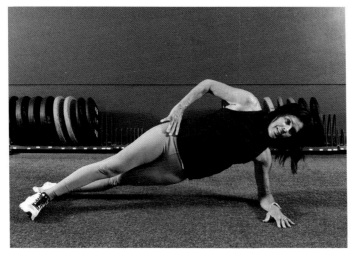

FIGURE 9.6   Side plank.

HOLLOW HOLD

Flip a plank over and you have a hollow hold, which is way harder than it looks. It's also one of the best core-strengthening exercises you can do. This is a very simple movement that can so easily be done wrong, so pay attention to the cues in the description. This is not just about lifting your arms and legs. There's a lot more going on!

Position

Lie on your back and reach your arms overhead, keeping your legs straight and resting on the floor (figure 9.7a).

Movement

Lift your head, shoulder blades (not just your arms), and legs off the floor at the same time while actively pushing your back into the floor as you contract your abs (figure 9.7b). Relax your shoulders and neck, keeping all the tension in your core. Hold the position for the prescribed time.

PRO CUE: Visualize making your body into a shape like a banana.

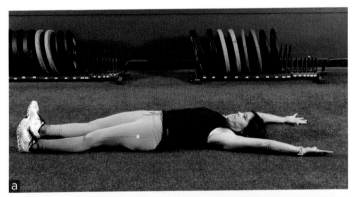

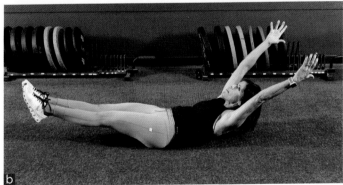

FIGURE 9.7   Hollow hold.

HANGING HOLLOW HOLD

This exercise is a progression from the hollow hold on the floor. It's also a first step to being able to do a pull-up. Hanging from the bar is one of the best positions for activating the core, as it decompresses the spine. It also provides a stretch for the shoulders in a full range of motion.

Position

Hang from a bar with your hands about shoulder-width apart and palms facing away from you in an overhand grip.

Movement

Think about pulling your shoulder blades down (doing the opposite of a shrug) while engaging your core in a hollow hold position (figure 9.8). Hold for 20 seconds, gradually working up to 60 seconds.

> **PRO CUE:** Visualize moving your armpits and hips toward each other. Keep your shoulders away from your ears!

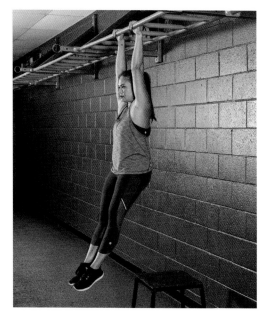

FIGURE 9.8   Hanging hollow hold.

CABLE HALF-KNEELING ANTI-ROTATION PRESS

We use the half-kneeling position often at Results Fitness for several reasons. In the half-kneeling position, it's easier to learn how to align your pelvis and rib cage, which is the most efficient position to stabilize your core and keep your back healthy. You're also getting a hip flexor stretch on the back leg. The position also mimics being on one leg with less stability demands than standing, helping to improve balance as you progress eventually to a standing position. In this exercise, you'll be resisting movement to stabilize your trunk while you move your arms.

Position

Stand sideways to a cable machine with the cable at waist height and your feet hip-width apart. Grab one handle with both hands. Lower the inside knee to the floor to come into a half-kneeling position and pull the cable handle close to your chest (figure 9.9a). The knee on the floor should be stacked underneath the hip, with both hips and shoulders squared forward, your chest proud, and your back straight. You'll be facing sideways to the cable machine with your inside knee on the floor and the front lower leg vertical in front of you.

Movement

Keeping your body stable and your shoulders down, press the handle straight out in front of you as you extend your elbows, feeling the pull from the cable machine forcing you to brace your core to stabilize (figure 9.9b). Hold the extended position for a few seconds before bending your elbows to return to the start position. Repeat for the number of reps and then switch sides. You can also perform this exercise in a tall-kneeling position: both knees on the ground.

> **PRO CUE:** Imagine the handle being a laser that could cut the body into an equal left and right half.

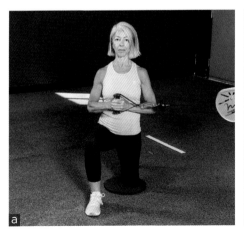 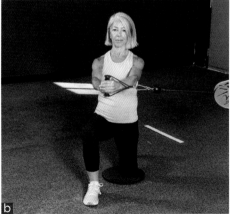

FIGURE 9.9 Cable half-kneeling anti-rotation press.

CABLE ROPE HALF-KNEELING CHOP

We encourage the half-kneeling position for several reasons. In the half-kneeling position, it's easier to learn how to align your pelvis and rib cage, which is the most efficient position to stabilize your core and keep your back from being strained. You're also stretching the hip flexor on the back leg. It also mimics being on one leg with less stability demands than standing, helping to improve balance as you progress eventually to a standing position.

Position

Stand sideways to a cable machine, your feet hip-width apart, with the cable at the top position on the machine. Using a triceps rope works best for this exercise so you can grab the ends with both hands. Lower the outside knee to the floor so you are in a half-kneeling position. The knee on the floor should be stacked underneath the hip, with both hips and shoulders squared forward, your chest proud, and your back straight. The shin of the front leg is vertical, and your arms are straight with your hands grasping the rope overhead toward the cable machine (figure 9.10a).

Movement

Keeping your arms straight, pull the cable across your body diagonally down to the opposite side in line with your hip (figure 9.10b). Your eyes will follow your hands while you maintain a tall posture, stabilize your trunk, and keep your shoulders and hips stacked. Pause, then return to the start position with control. Repeat for the desired number of repetitions, then repeat on the other side.

> **PRO CUE:** Visualize making yourself one inch taller that you truly are while performing this movement to improve your posture.

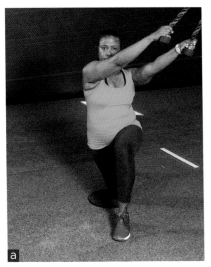 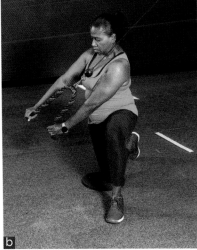

FIGURE 9.10 Cable rope half-kneeling chop.

CABLE HALF-KNEELING LIFT

Rather than the chopping movement you performed in the last exercise, this exercise mimics a lifting motion. Again, in the half-kneeling position, it's easier to learn how to align your pelvis and rib cage, which is the most efficient position to stabilize your core and keep your back from being strained. You're also stretching the hip flexor on the back leg. And it mimics being on one leg with less of a stability demand than standing, helping to improve balance as you progress eventually to a standing position.

Position

Stand sideways to a cable machine, your feet hip-width apart, with the cable at the bottom position. Using a triceps rope works best for this exercise so you can grab the ends with both hands. Lower your inside knee to the floor to come into a half-kneeling position. The knee on the floor should be stacked underneath the hip, with both hips and shoulders squared forward, your chest proud, and your back straight. The shin of the front leg is vertical and your arms are straight. Hold the rope near the hip closest to the cable machine (figure 9.11*a*).

Movement

Keeping your arms straight, pull the cable across your body and diagonally up to the opposite side overhead (figure 9.11*b*). Your eyes will follow your hands while you maintain a tall posture, stabilizing your trunk and keeping your shoulders and hips stacked. Pause, then return to the start position under control. Repeat for the desired number of repetitions, then repeat on the other side.

> **PRO CUE:** Visualize making yourself one inch taller that you truly are while performing this movement to improve your posture.

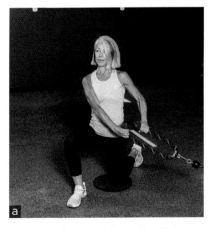
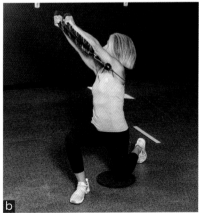

FIGURE 9.11   Cable half-kneeling lift.

CABLE HORIZONTAL WOOD CHOP

Many exercise programs neglect the transverse plane or the movement of rotating your body in one direction and then the other. This exercise is a progression from the half-kneeling chops and lifts; now you're ready to take it to a standing position to perform wood chops using your whole body. This exercise works your entire kinetic chain using several muscles.

Position

Stand sideways to a cable machine with the cable at hip height. Grab the handle with both hands, your outside hand on the bottom. Step away from the machine until the cable has tension. Your arms are straight and your hands are positioned in the direction of the machine (figure 9.12*a*). Your feet should be wider than shoulder-width apart in a stable standing position.

Movement

Bending the knee closest to the cable machine, keep your arms straight as you pull the cable across your body. Shift your weight to bend the outside knee as you pull the cable, finishing with the handle in line with your outside hip (figure 9.12*b*). Keep your eyes on your hands as you perform the movement. Return to the start position under control. Repeat for the desired number of reps, then switch sides.

> **PRO CUE:** Before you initiate the movement, brace the torso as if to take a punch in the gut.

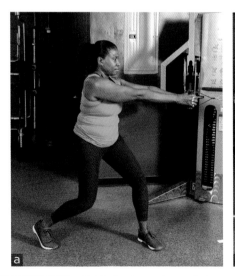 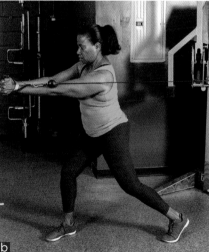

FIGURE 9.12   Cable horizontal wood chop.

SANDBAG DEAD BUG ALTERNATING-LEG REACH

This exercise uses a sandbag to create tension in the core while you actively move your legs. You could also use a stiff band or towel if you don't have a sandbag.

Position

Lie on your back, holding the sandbag with both hands, your arms extended straight up and positioned over your chest. Press your lower back into the ground and lift both legs off the floor so that the hips and knees are at 90-degree angles (figure 9.13a).

Movement

Imagine pulling the bag apart as you engage the lats and straighten and lower one leg until it is fully extended, hovering just above the floor (figure 9.13b). Keep pressing your lower back to the floor throughout the exercise. Return the leg to the start position and repeat with the opposite leg. Do not release the tension of the upper body during the exercise. Repeat for the desired number of repetitions, alternating each leg.

> **PRO CUE:** Imagine that there is a thick exercise band underneath the small of your back and that someone is trying to pull the band out from under you. Press the low back down toward the ground to prevent it from being pulled out as you perform this exercise.

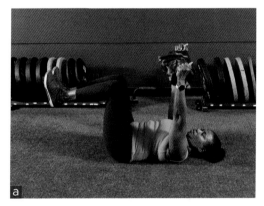 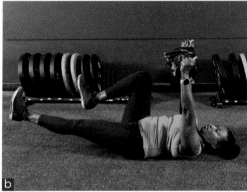

FIGURE 9.13   Sandbag dead bug alternating-leg reach.

SANDBAG FULL DEAD BUG

This exercise progresses the dead bug with leg reach to include a reach with the upper body as well, creating a cross-body core connection with the sandbag. You could also use a stiff band or towel if you don't have a sandbag. You'll be actively bracing and stabilizing your core while moving both your upper body and your lower body. This is an extremely challenging exercise when it is done with intent. Pay attention to the cues.

Position

Lie on your back, holding the sandbag with both hands and extending your arms straight up, positioning them over your chest. Press your lower back into the ground and lift both legs off the floor so that the hips and knees are at 90-degree angles (figure 9.14a).

Movement

Imagine pulling the bag apart as you engage the lats. Reach with one arm back to extend overhead, pulling the bag with you while straightening and lowering the opposite leg until it is fully extended and hovering above the floor (figure 9.14b). Keep pressing your lower back to the floor throughout the exercise. Return to the start position and repeat with the opposite arm and leg. Do not release the tension of the upper body on the bag during the exercise.

PRO CUE: Keep the tension on the bag during the movement to keep it from sagging.

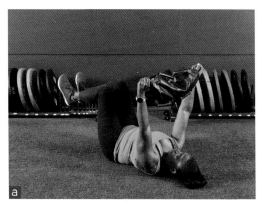
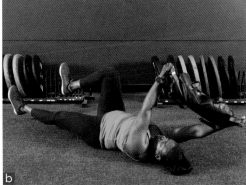

FIGURE 9.14   Sandbag full dead bug.

SUSPENSION TRAINER PRONE JACKKNIFE

It's time to really challenge your core by trying out some unstable positions using a suspension trainer. You'll be in the plank position once again, except this time your feet will be suspended in a suspension trainer, and you'll perform a dynamic movement with the hips and knees while keeping your trunk stable.

Position

With a suspension trainer secured overhead, adjust the straps so that when you are standing next to the straps, the bottoms of the foot cradles are halfway between your ankles and knees at the midpoint of your shins. Place both feet in the straps. Position yourself in the top of a push-up, with your arms supporting your weight (figure 9.15a). Your head, shoulders, and hips are all in one straight line, your hands stacked under your shoulders. Your legs are straight with your feet in the straps and your toes pulled toward the shins.

Movement

Maintaining a plank position with a stable trunk, tuck your knees in under your body (figure 9.15b), then return to the start position. Keep your upper body, from the hips up, as still as possible as you stabilize your core during the movement. Repeat tucking your knees in, then straightening for the desired number of reps.

PRO CUE: Maintain the level alignment of the head, shoulders, and hips, as if a dowel rod on your back was touching the back of the head, the upper back, and hips.

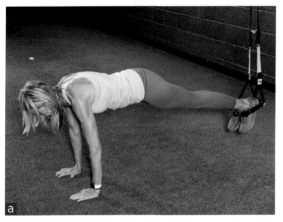
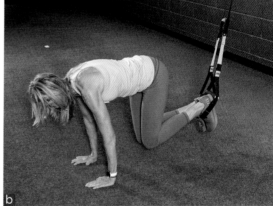

FIGURE 9.15   Suspension trainer prone jackknife.

CHAPTER 10

UPPER BODY

Strengthening your upper body to stand tall and keeping your shoulders and upper back strong and healthy will give you improved posture as you age so you won't look like a rounded-over, hunched old lady. Don't be afraid to lift heavy with your upper body to build some muscle.

INCLINE PUSH-UP

If you've always done "girl push-ups" or push-ups on your knees, it's time to start challenging yourself to do real push-ups. Start with these incline push-ups and eventually work your way down until you're doing a push-up on the floor. Push-ups work your upper body, including your shoulders and chest, and they are also a core-strengthening exercise because you are in a plank position.

Position

Place your hands on a sturdy step, bar, bench, or wall (easiest version). Walk your feet out until your weight is on your feet and hands (figure 10.1a). Your heels will come off the floor. Your spine should be in a straight line with your head, upper back, and tailbone.

Movement

Bend at your elbows to lower your chest toward the step, bar, bench, or wall, keeping your body in a straight line and your abdominals engaged (figure 10.1b). Be careful not to let your back arch or sag and keep your hips from sticking up. Lower yourself until your shoulders go just below your elbows, then return to the start position, keeping your body in a plank position during the entire movement. Repeat for the desired number of reps.

> **PRO CUE:** Lead the movement with the logo on your shirt rather than your face. Leading with the face often results in a chicken neck and the false perception that you are going lower than you actually are!

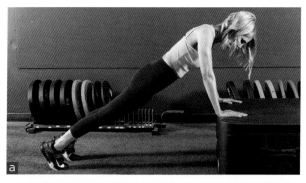

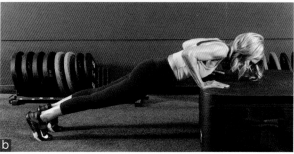

FIGURE 10.1 Incline push-up.

PUSH-UP

You've been performing incline push-ups, and now it's time to give full push-ups a try. Push-ups not only work your upper body including your shoulders and chest but also strengthen your core while you are in a plank position.

Position

Lie on your abdomen and place your hands in line with your chin just outside of shoulder-width. Tuck your toes under to be ready to put weight on your feet (figure 10.2*a*). Your spine should be in a straight line, with your head, upper back, and tailbone in alignment.

Movement

Keeping your body straight, press yourself up to a top plank position with your abdominals engaged (figure 10.2*b*). Be careful not to let your back arch or sag and keep your hips from sticking up. Lower yourself until your shoulders go just below your elbows, then return to the start position, keeping your body in a plank position during the entire movement. Repeat for the desired number of reps. As you are able to perform the reps with good form, you can add load by having a training partner or coach carefully place a plate or a sandbag on your back.

> PRO CUE: **Lead the movement with the logo on your shirt rather than your face.**

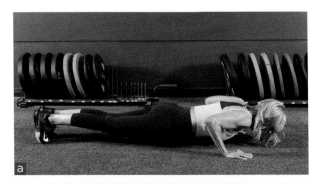

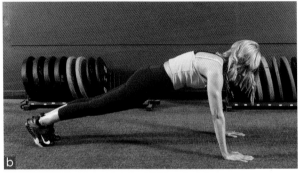

FIGURE 10.2 Push-up.

CABLE HALF-KNEELING ONE-ARM ROW

We use the half-kneeling position for several reasons. It's easier to learn how to align your pelvis and rib cage, which is the most efficient position to stabilize your core and keep your back healthy. You're getting a hip flexor stretch on the back leg. It mimics being on one leg with less of a stability demand than standing, helping to improve balance as you progress eventually to a standing position.

Position

Stand in front of a cable machine with the cable at waist height, your feet hip-width apart, and the cable an arm's distance away. Lower yourself onto one knee with your front shin vertical. The knee on the floor should be stacked underneath the hip, with both the hips and shoulders squared forward, your chest proud, and your back straight. Grab the cable with the same arm as the knee that is on the ground (figure 10.3*a*).

Movement

Using your upper back, pull the cable toward your waist, bringing your elbow toward your side (figure 10.3*b*). As your elbow grazes the side of your body, continue to pull until it is just past your midline, keeping your elbow in close to your body and your shoulder down and back. Pause and then reverse the movement with control. Repeat for the desired number of repetitions, then switch sides.

> **PRO CUE:** Initiate the movement by leading with the shoulder blade. Think of stretching the front of your shirt when the elbow is back.

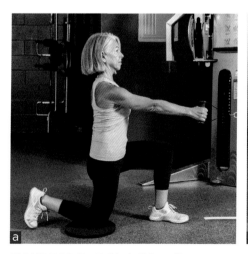 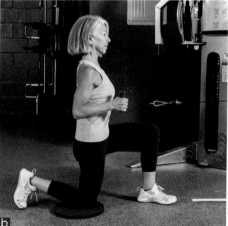

FIGURE 10.3 Cable half-kneeling one-arm row.

CABLE ONE-LEG ONE-ARM ROW

After you've spent time in the half-kneeling position and learned the stacked position with your hips engaging your core to keep your trunk stable, you're ready to challenge your balance by standing on one leg.

Position

Stand in front of a cable machine with the cable at chest height, your feet hip-width apart, and the cable an arm's distance away. Shift your weight to one leg. Your hips and shoulders are squared ahead, your chest is proud, and your back is straight. Grab the cable with the opposite arm from the standing leg, and fully extend your arm in front of you (figure 10.4a).

Movement

Using your upper back, pull the cable toward your waist, bringing your elbow toward your side (figure 10.4b). As your elbow grazes the side of your body, continue to pull until it is past your midline, keeping your elbow in close to your body and your shoulder down and back. Pause and then reverse the movement with control. Repeat for the desired number of repetitions, then switch sides.

> PRO CUE: Initiate the movement by leading with the shoulder blade. Think of stretching the front of your shirt at when the elbow is back.

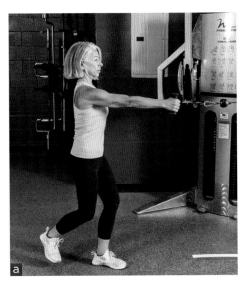 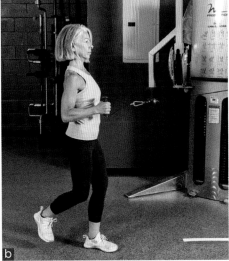

FIGURE 10.4   Cable one-leg one-arm row.

CABLE TALL-KNEELING NEUTRAL-GRIP PULL-DOWN

Performing a pull-down from a kneeling position instead of a seated one opens your hips to an extended position, stretching the hip flexors and aligning your pelvis and rib cage. This is the most efficient position to stabilize your core and keep your back healthy.

Position

With the handles of the cable machine at a width just outside of shoulder width at the top position, kneel directly below the handles. Grasp the handles with the arms extended overhead and palms facing each other (figure 10.5*a*). Your shoulders, hips and knees should all be stacked in a vertical line, with your core engaged and your back flat.

Movement

Using your upper-back muscles, pull the handles toward you as you bring your elbows toward the sides of your body (figure 10.5*b*). Pull your shoulder blades down and back, as if putting them in your back pockets. As you're pulling down, lift your chest without hyperextending the lower back. Pause and then reverse the movement with control. Repeat for the desired number of reps.

> **PRO CUE:** Keep the shoulders "out of the ears" at the bottom position.

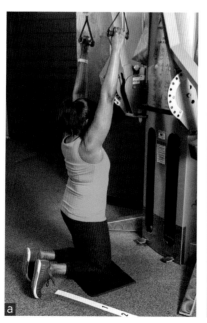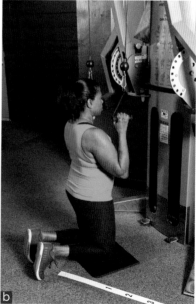

FIGURE 10.5   Cable tall-kneeling neutral-grip pull-down.

CABLE TALL-KNEELING OVERHAND-GRIP PULL-DOWN

Turning your hands to face away from you makes the pull-down movement more challenging because the biceps will be less involved and the lats will be more involved as you perform the movement.

Position

With the handles of the cable machine outside of shoulder width at the top position, kneel directly below the cable attachment, holding the handles with your arms extended overhead and your palms facing away from you (figure 10.6*a*). Your shoulders, hips, and knees should all be stacked in a vertical line, with your core engaged and your back flat.

Movement

Using your upper-back muscles, pull the handles toward you as you bring your elbows toward the sides of your body (figure 10.6*b*). Pull your shoulder blades down and back, as if putting them in your back pockets. As you're pulling down, lift your chest without hyperextending your lower back. Pause and then reverse the movement with control. Repeat for the desired number of reps.

PRO CUE: Keep the shoulders "out of the ears" at the bottom position.

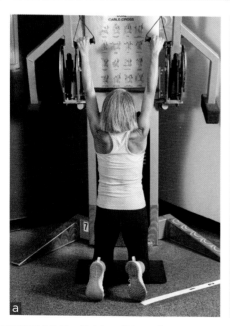
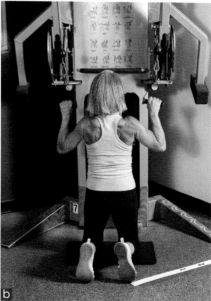

FIGURE 10.6   Cable tall-kneeling overhand-grip pull-down.

CABLE TALL-KNEELING UNDERHAND-GRIP PULL-DOWN

The last variation of a pull-down is a medium grip. The neutral grip is easiest, the overhand grip is hardest, and the underhand grip is in between. This means you can add more weight than the overhand version.

Position

With the handles of the cable machine at shoulder-width at the top position, kneel directly below the cable attachment, holding the handles extended overhead with your palms facing your body (figure 10.7a). Shoulders, hips, and knees should all be stacked in a vertical line with your core engaged and your back flat.

Movement

Using your upper-back muscles, pull the handles toward you as you bring your elbows toward the sides of your body (figure 10.7b). Pull your shoulder blades down and back, as if putting them in your back pockets. As you're pulling down, lift your chest. Pause and then reverse the movement with control. Repeat for the desired number of reps.

> **PRO CUE:** Keep the shoulders "out of the ears" at the bottom position.

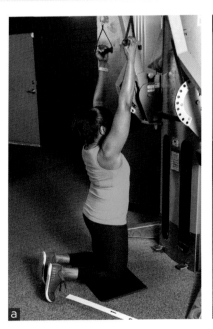 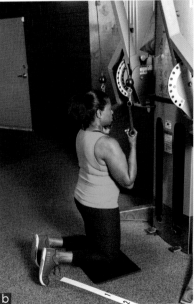

FIGURE 10.7   Cable tall-kneeling underhand-grip pull-down.

DUMBBELL THREE-POINT NEUTRAL-GRIP ROW

Tall posture and a strong back are crucial to staying young and fit. Performing a row using a dumbbell in a bent-over position fires up your lats and entire posterior chain.

Position

Hold a dumbbell in your right hand. Stand with a bench in front of you and bend over to place your left hand on the bench. Your feet should be shoulder-width apart and directly under the hips, and your back is flat with your head, spine, and tailbone in alignment. Extend the arm holding the dumbbell so that it hangs straight down (figure 10.8a).

Movement

Pull the dumbbell toward you, bringing your elbow toward your body in a rowing motion (figure 10.8b). Imagine pulling with your shoulder blade while maintaining a neutral position with your back. Be careful not to shrug your shoulder up as you perform the movement. Lower the weight and repeat for the desired number of reps, then switch sides.

> PRO CUE: Imagine that you are wearing a hooded sweatshirt with pockets and pull the dumbbell into position beside the pocket.

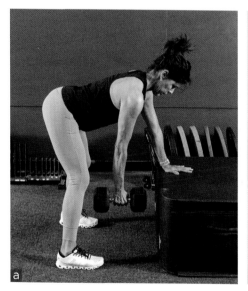 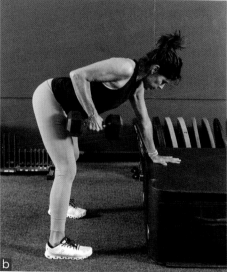

FIGURE 10.8   Dumbbell three-point neutral-grip row.

DUMBBELL TWO-POINT ROW

This progression of the bent-over dumbbell row removes the hand on the bench. You'll work just a bit harder.

Position

Hold a dumbbell in one hand. Stand with your feet shoulder-width apart and hinge forward at the hips to about a 45-degree angle, extending your arm to let the dumbbell hang straight down (figure 10.9a). Your feet should be directly under your hips, and your back should be flat, with your head, spine, and tailbone in alignment. Your other arm can be behind your back or on your hip.

Movement

Pull the dumbbell toward you, bringing your elbow toward your body in a rowing motion (figure 10.9b). Imagine pulling with your shoulder blade while maintaining a neutral position with your back. Be careful not to shrug your shoulder as you perform the movement. Lower the weight and repeat for the desired number of reps, then switch sides.

> **PRO CUE:** Imagine that you are wearing a hooded sweatshirt with pockets and pull the dumbbell into position beside the pocket. Also, maintain some space between the upper arm and the torso at the finish; this will allow the shoulder blade to move properly.

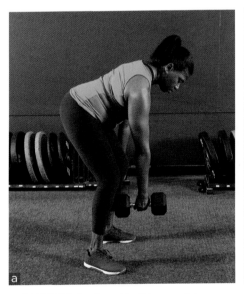 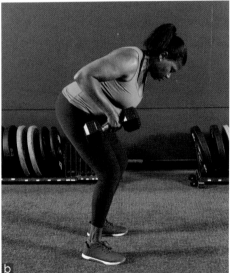

FIGURE 10.9 Dumbbell two-point row.

SUSPENSION TRAINER INVERTED NEUTRAL-GRIP ROW

The inverted row is the opposite of the push-up: You perform a rowing movement in the plank position, working not only the upper back but also the entire body. You'll feel your legs, butt, core, and upper body working.

Position

With a suspension trainer strap secured overhead, the handles hanging at chest height, and your feet hip-width apart, hold on to the handles with your palms facing each other. Lean back until your arms are fully extended (figure 10.10*a*). Your body should be in a straight line, as if in a plank position—shoulders, hips, and knees all in alignment. The position of your feet will determine how easy or hard the exercise is: Walk your feet toward or even past the anchor point to make it more difficult (your body is more horizontal) or further away from the anchor point to make it easier. Take note of where you have your feet so that you can progress the exercise as you get stronger.

Movement

Pull your elbows toward your body and lift your body toward the anchor point while maintaining the plank position and keeping the core engaged (figure 10.10*b*). Keep your shoulders down and back using your upper back and lats to perform the exercise without shrugging. Pause at the top position, then slowly return. Repeat for the desired number of reps.

> **PRO CUE:** Initiate the movement by leading with the shoulder blades, not just by bending the elbows. Think of stretching the front of your shirt at the top position.

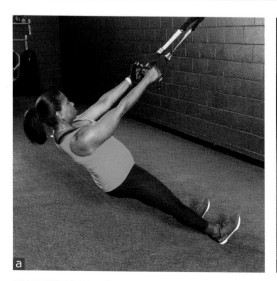
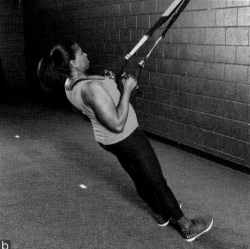

FIGURE 10.10   Suspension trainer inverted neutral-grip row.

DUMBBELL HALF-KNEELING ONE-ARM OVERHEAD PRESS

The half-kneeling position makes it easier to learn to properly align your pelvis and rib cage, which is the most efficient position to stabilize your core and keep your back healthy. This position also gives you a hip flexor stretch on the back leg. A half-kneeling position is more stable than a standing position on one leg, helping you improve balance as you progress to a standing position.

Position

Stand with feet hip-width apart. Lower yourself onto one knee with your front shin vertical. The knee on the floor should be stacked underneath the hip, with both hips and shoulders squared forward, your chest proud, and your back straight. Hold a dumbbell at shoulder height in the same arm as the leg that is on the floor ready to press overhead (figure 10.11*a*).

Movement

Keeping your trunk stabilized, push the dumbbell straight up overhead until your arm is fully extended (figure 10.11*b*). Pause and then reverse the movement with control. Repeat for the desired number of reps, then switch sides for both the leg and arm.

> **PRO CUE:** Finish the top of the movement with the arm vertical at 12 o'clock as viewed from both the front or back and the sides.

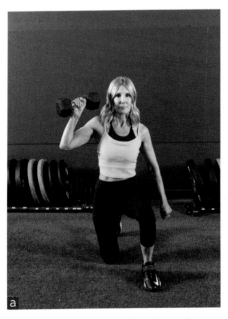 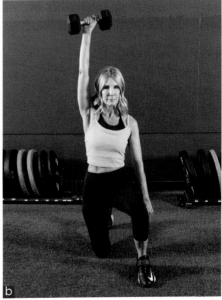

FIGURE 10.11   Dumbbell half-kneeling one-arm overhead press.

DUMBBELL INCLINE BENCH PRESS

Lying on a bench and pressing dumbbells up to perform a simple dumbbell bench press is one of my favorite exercises because you can progress quickly and feel what it is like to get strong. There's no better feeling than knowing you can press a 30-, 40-, or even 50-pound dumbbell.

Position

Lie on your back on an incline bench, holding a dumbbell in each hand. Your feet are flat on the floor, and your back is in a neutral position on the bench. The dumbbells will be at shoulder height, with your palms facing your feet (figure 10.13*a*).

Movement

Push the dumbbells straight up until your arms are fully extended (figure 10.13*b*). Keep your feet flat on the floor throughout the entire movement. Repeat for the desired number of reps, then switch sides.

> **PRO CUE:** At the bottom of the movement, the upper arm will be at an angle of approximately 45 degrees from the torso.

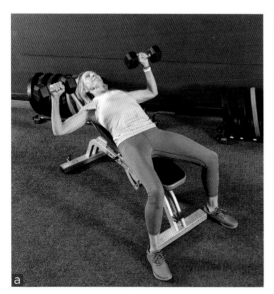 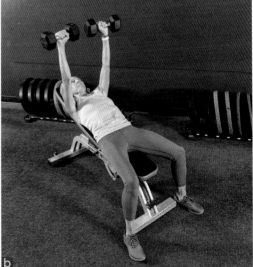

FIGURE 10.12 Dumbbell incline bench press.

DUMBBELL ONE-ARM BENCH PRESS

This exercise takes the old-school dumbbell bench press to another level as you will perform it one arm at a time. This forces your core to engage: With weight on one side, you'll feel your abs working to stabilize your body, turning it into more than just an upper-body chest exercise.

Position

Lie on your back on a bench, holding a dumbbell in one hand. Your feet are flat on the floor, and your back is in a neutral position on the bench. The dumbbell will be at shoulder height, and your palm is facing your feet (figure 10.13a).

Movement

Push the dumbbell straight up until your arm is fully extended (figure 10.13b). You'll feel your body leaning toward the weighted arm, and you'll need to engage your core to stabilize yourself on the bench. Keep your feet flat on the floor throughout the entire movement. Repeat for the desired number of reps, then switch sides.

> **PRO CUE:** At the bottom of the movement, the upper arm will be at an angle of approximately 45 degrees from the torso.

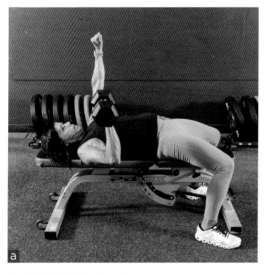
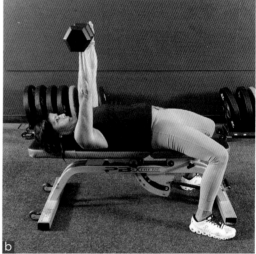

FIGURE 10.13   Dumbbell one-arm bench press.

CHAPTER 11

LOWER BODY

Don't be afraid to lift heavy with your lower body. By lifting heavy, you'll create a demand on the big muscles that will help you to build your metabolism, drive your anabolic hormones up, and get strong and fit as you age. This chapter is full of fantastic lower-body exercises.

KETTLEBELL GOBLET SQUAT

This exercise helps you learn the proper biomechanics of the squat movement. By counterbalancing your weight while holding a kettlebell in front of you, you'll find performing a squat with a full range of motion much easier.

Position

Stand with your feet approximately shoulder-width apart and your toes pointed slightly out. Hold a kettlebell at chest height with both hands, tucking your elbows in and pulling as if you are trying to rip the handle of the kettlebell apart to engage your lats. Keep your shoulders down and your chest proud and tall (figure 11.1a).

Movement

Bend at the knees and hips into a full squat position while keeping your feet firmly planted on the floor and your knees over your toes (figure 11.1b). Maintain a proud posture and continue to create tension while holding the kettlebell. Keep your lower back from rounding. At the bottom position, your elbows will be inside your knees and your chest will be upright. Engage the glute muscles to return to the standing position. Repeat for the desired number of reps.

> **PRO CUE:** Visualize gripping the ground slightly with your feet just before initiating the descent into the squat and continue to grip during the movement. This will help keep the joints involved in the squat in proper alignment.

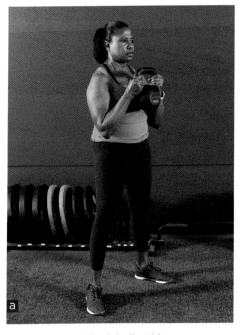 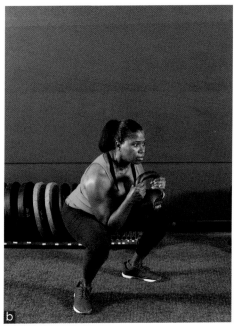

FIGURE 11.1 Kettlebell goblet squat.

GOBLET SPLIT SQUAT

Once you've moved out of the base phase and have mastered some of the fundamental movements of the squat, it's time to progress to a split stance. The split stance creates some instability and puts more demands on the core. A split stance also makes the movement more difficult because of the increased demands on the working leg, while the opposite leg is in an active stretch. This movement transfers to activities such as running, helping to create more efficient movement and strength.

Position

Stand with your feet shoulder-width apart, holding a kettlebell at chest height in both hands, your shoulders back and chest proud. Step forward about 3 feet with one foot (figure 11.2a). Your body weight should be evenly distributed across both feet. Grip the handles of the kettlebell with tension to engage your lats and upper back.

Movement

Bend your front knee as you lower the back knee toward the ground until it grazes the ground (figure 11.2b). Keep your torso upright and your shoulders down, and continue gripping the kettlebell to engage your lats and upper back. Once you've reached the end of your range of motion, drive through the front foot to return to the top staggered position. Repeat for the desired number of repetitions, then switch sides.

> **PRO CUE:** Keep the belt line level and square front to back and side to side while performing this movement. It is helpful to think of it as a "moving" half-kneeling vertical plank.

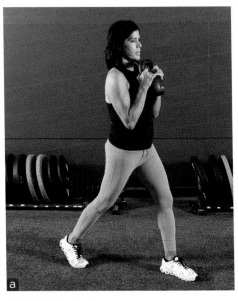 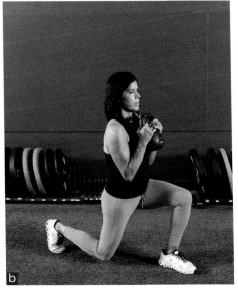

FIGURE 11.2   Goblet split squat.

REAR FOOT ELEVATED SPLIT SQUAT

This is one of the most difficult yet most effective exercises in the final phase of the Age Strong program. Start with your body weight, then hold dumbbells or a kettlebell as you master the movement.

Position

Stand with a bench (or a single-leg squat stand) behind you. Put one foot on the bench and the other 2 to 3 feet in front of the bench (figure 11.3*a*). You'll be in a modified split squat position with your back leg raised, placing more demand on your front leg. This position also challenges your balance and core stability. As you get stronger, add weight by holding a dumbbell in each hand at your sides or a kettlebell in both hands in front of your chest (goblet position).

Movement

With most of your weight on your front leg, bend your front knee until your front thigh is about parallel to the floor and your back knee grazes the floor or a pad (figure 11.3*b*). If you are unable to lower your back knee to the floor or a pad, you may need to regress the exercise to a lunge until you're able to perform it with a full range of motion. Keep your body weight on your front leg; do not sit back to put weight on your back leg. Pause in the lowered position, then drive through the front leg to return to the start position. Repeat for the desired number of repetitions, then switch sides.

> **PRO CUE:** Visualize wearing a knee pad on the back leg and imagine lowering the knee pad almost straight down to the floor as you perform the movement.

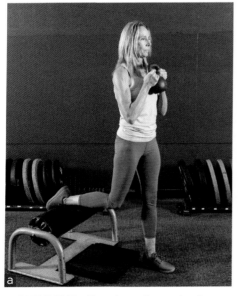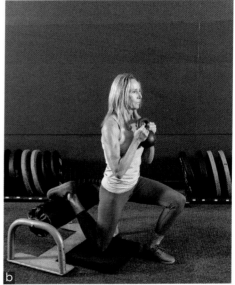

FIGURE 11.3   Rear foot elevated split squat.

FRONT SQUAT

Front squats force you to have good form. Because the barbell is on the front of your shoulders, you must keep your body upright with your elbows high and maintain good form with your back as you perform the squat or the bar will fall forward. The front squat forces you to use your upper-back muscles to keep your body from tipping forward. Start with a barbell with no weight plates on it, and then add weight as you master the movement and your form.

Position

With your arms straight in front of you, walk up to the bar in a squat rack until the bar is lightly touching your neck. Place the bar as high on your collarbone as comfortable. The bar will rest on a shelf you'll create with your shoulders. Grip the bar with your hands as close to your shoulders as is comfortable with your elbows pointing directly forward. Lift the bar, step back from the squat rack, and stand with your feet shoulder-width apart and your feet straight or slightly angled out (figure 11.4a).

Movement

Keeping your torso upright, bend at the knees and hips to squat as deeply as you can (figure 11.4b), then return to the start position. Your knees should stay an equal distance apart and your elbows should stay high, keeping the barbell secure on the shelf created by your shoulders. The downward motion should exactly mirror the upward one.

> PRO CUE: Imagine that you have laser pointers coming out of your elbows at the top of the movement. Keep those laser pointers projected straight in front you as you perform the movement.

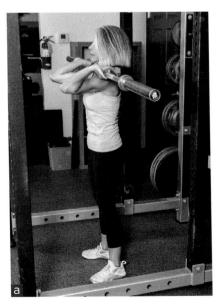
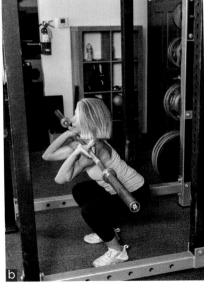

FIGURE 11.4   Front squat.

STEP-UP

An important movement to train as you age is stepping up and stepping down. Being able to go up and down stairs will keep you in the game of life. That's why in the base phase you'll learn how to do a proper step-up, making sure you're engaging the right muscles and keeping your knees strong and healthy.

Position

Stand facing a step or bench at about knee height and place one foot on top of the step (figure 11.5a). Stand with a tall, proud chest and keep your shoulders down.

Movement

Lean your body weight onto the foot on the step and drive through that leg to lift your body to the top of the step (figure 11.5b). Do your best to not push off the trailing leg and keep it from touching the step. Lower with control to the start position. Pause at the bottom. Repeat for the desired number of repetitions, then switch sides.

Increase the height of the step as you get stronger until it's at hip height. You can then add a dumbbell in each hand or another load.

> **PRO CUE:** Keep the torso engaged and vertical while performing this movement. The belt line should stay relatively level front to back and side to side.

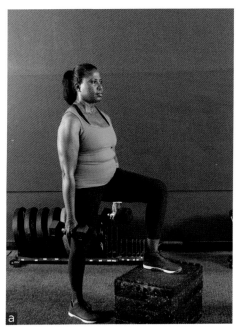 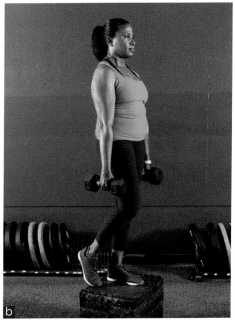

FIGURE 11.5 Step-up.

SANDBAG STAGGERED-STANCE RDL

This exercise introduces one of the fundamental movements of a strength training program: the one-leg hip hinge. With a proper hip hinge, you'll work your posterior chain (all the muscles in the back of your leg and hip), which will make you much more efficient and potentially less likely to get injured. Completely balancing on one leg can be tricky, which is why I first introduce this staggered-stance position for you to learn the movement.

Using a sandbag while learning this exercise teaches you to pull apart the bag, engaging the lats and upper back. This helps connect the upper and lower body to work as one integrated machine. If you don't have a sandbag, you can use a barbell.

Position

Stand with your feet shoulder-width apart. Hold the sandbag in front of you with your arms extended. Hold the parallel handles and pulling them apart to engage your lats and upper back. Step back with one foot until the foot is in line with the heel of the other foot (figure 11.6a).

Movement

Hinge forward at the hips, reaching your hips back as you lower the bag along the front of your legs (figure 11.6b). Continue to engage your lats and upper back by pulling apart the handles of the bag as you bend, keeping your back from rounding. You can place the bag on a high step as a marker of how far to bend. Just before you get to the point where you can no longer keep your spine in a neutral position, return to the standing position by contracting the glutes, again keeping the path of the sandbag right along the front of the legs. Repeat for the desired number of repetitions, then switch the legs.

> **PRO CUE:** Imagine that you are standing with your hips in the center of a compass facing north. Visualize pushing your back pockets straight back south.

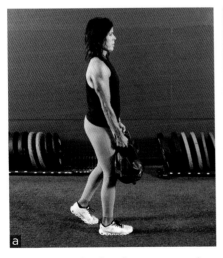 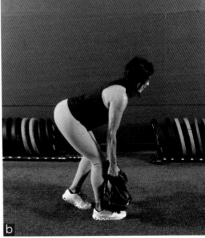

FIGURE 11.6   Sandbag staggered-stance RDL.

KETTLEBELL STAGGERED-STANCE RDL

After mastering the hip hinge movement using a sandbag, you'll switch it out for a kettlebell in one hand. This creates an offset load and increases the demand on the core. You also can progress the load to a heavier weight as you get stronger.

Position

Stand with the kettlebell in one hand, your feet about hip-width apart. With the foot on the same side as the kettlebell, step back so that foot is in line with the heel of the other foot (figure 11.7*a*). Your weight is on the leg opposite the kettlebell.

Movement

Hinge forward at the hips, reaching your hips back as you lower the kettlebell along the front of your body in line with your front leg (figure 11.7*b*). Engage your lats and upper back as you hinge forward, keeping your back from rounding. Once you get to where you can no longer keep your spine in a neutral position (it is not a bad idea to have a training partner or coach tell you when), return to a standing position by contracting the glutes. The entire time, keep the kettlebell along the front of the body in line with the front leg as if you are setting it down on the inside of the front leg.

> **PRO CUE:** Imagine that you are standing with your hips in the center of a compass facing north. Visualize pushing your back pockets straight back south.

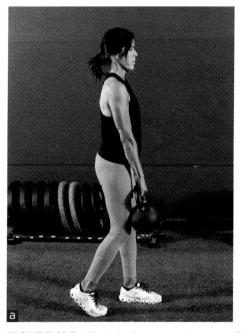 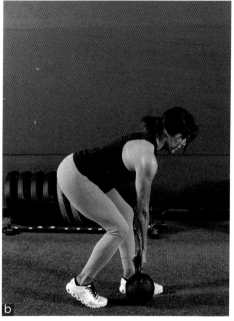

FIGURE 11.7   Kettlebell staggered-stance RDL.

SANDBAG SLIDER ONE-LEG RDL

As you move into phase three, the Stronger Phase, you'll progress the exercises even further. Now, you'll use a slider for your back foot to make your front leg work even more, increasing the demand on that leg to improve your strength to a new level while also adding a further demand on your core. You'll go back to using the sandbag with this progressed version for this phase, performing a higher number of reps as you get stronger.

Position

Stand with your feet shoulder-width apart and a slider under one foot. Hold the sandbag in front of you with your arms extended (figure 11.8*a*). Hold the parallel handles and pull them apart, engaging your lats and upper back.

Movement

Hinge forward at the hips, reaching your hips back as you lower the bag along the front of your legs and slide one leg to reach back as far as you can. Maintain a neutral spine as you load the front leg (figure 11.8*b*). Continue to engage your lats and upper back by pulling apart the handles of the bag as you hinge, keeping your back from rounding. Once you get to where you can no longer keep your spine in a neutral position, return to standing by contracting the glutes and loading the front leg as you slide the back leg in. Throughout the movement, keep the sandbag in line with the front leg. Repeat for the desired number of reps, then switch sides.

> **PRO CUE:** Keep the back leg straight and imagine just skimming the ground with the slider.

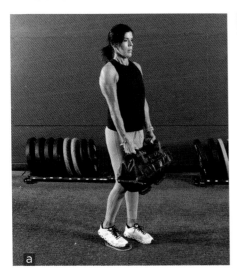
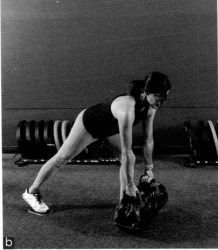

FIGURE 11.8   Sandbag slider one-leg RDL.

DUMBBELL ONE-LEG RDL

This is what you've been working up to: You've mastered the staggered stance and progressed to using a slider, and now you'll balance on one leg while performing a one-leg Romanian deadlift. This will fully load one leg while challenging your balance and stability to put your core to work. You'll use your entire posterior chain as well.

Position

Stand on one leg with a slight bend in the knee and the other leg hovering above the ground, holding a dumbbell in the opposite hand with the arm extended (figure 11.9a). Stand tall with a proud chest.

Movement

Balancing on one leg, hinge forward at the hips, reaching your hips back as you lower the dumbbell along the front of your body in line with your front leg to place it on the inside of your front leg (figure 11.9b). Your back foot will reach slightly behind you as you're reaching back with your hips while keeping your hips square. Engage your lats and upper back as you hinge forward, keeping your back from rounding. You can place the dumbbell on a box or step as a marker of how far to go if you're unable to reach the floor without rounding your back. Just before you get to the point where you can no longer keep your spine in a neutral position, return to a standing position by contracting the glutes.

> **PRO CUE:** Your stance leg (the stationary or working leg) must have a slight bend. This is essential to allow a posterior weight shift to occur. For your lifted leg, visualize leaving a footprint on the wall behind you as you lower yourself to the bottom of the hip hinge.

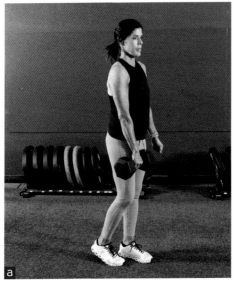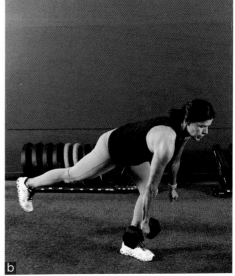

FIGURE 11.9   Dumbbell one-leg RDL.

KETTLEBELL DEADLIFT

If there is one exercise I recommend you master and get stronger at as you age, it's the deadlift. Being able to bend down and pick something up is a crucial task that many lose the ability to do as they age. It's also one of the best full-body exercises; as you hold the weight, you strengthen your upper and lower back, your legs, your core, and your arms. Using a kettlebell as you initially learn the deadlift movement will help you learn the fundamentals.

Position

Place the kettlebell between your heels with your feet outside of shoulder-width apart and slightly turned out. Keeping a proud chest showing the logo across the front of your T-shirt and your eyes focused on a spot about 7 to 10 feet in front of you, bend to grab the handle of the kettlebell with both hands without letting your heels come off the floor or rounding your back (figure 11.10*a*).

Movement

Grasping the handle of the kettlebell, think about sitting into your hips to pull the kettlebell straight up along your body. Keep your shoulders pulled down, your chest proud at the top, and your ribs down (figure 11.10*b*). Bend your knees and hips to lower the kettlebell back to the start position while maintaining a neutral spine and proud chest. Repeat for the desired number of repetitions.

> **PRO CUE:** Rather than yanking on the kettlebell with your back or arms, visualize connecting to the kettlebell and pushing your feet through the floor with patience as you hinge up.

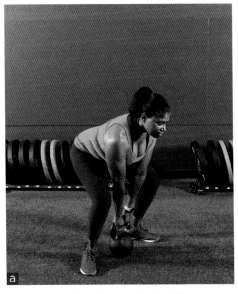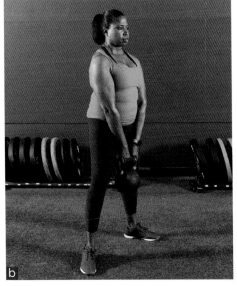

FIGURE 11.10   Kettlebell deadlift.

HIGH HEX BAR DEADLIFT

Using a barbell or hex bar (also commonly called a trap bar) helps you to master your form in the deadlift, because it keeps the bar's center of mass lined up with your base of support. Many clients typically deadlift with a hex bar instead of a barbell unless they are powerlifters. Once you can deadlift the 28 kilogram (62 lb) kettlebell, it's time to start using a barbell or hex bar.

A note on range of motion: Put Olympic-size plates (big plates) on the hex bar or barbell to provide the range of motion from the floor you want for this exercise. If you do not have 10-pound or 25-pound Olympic-size plates, you'll need to set the plates on a box or step to decrease the range of motion. If you use small-diameter plates, you'll go too low and most likely will not be able to keep your form. In addition, the hex bar has both high and low handles. Use the high handles to keep your range of motion at a level where you can maintain your form.

Position

Place two Olympic-size plates on the hex bar and use collars to secure them in place. Stand in the middle of the hex bar with a tall posture and grab the high handles. Sit into your hips, keeping your heels down and your feet planted on the floor and your spine in a neutral position (figure 11.11*a*). Your hips will be higher than your knees and lower than your shoulders when viewed from the side.

Movement

Push your feet into the ground to stand straight up while keeping your back in a neutral position (not rounded) as you lift (figure 11.11*b*). Pause at the top and then lower the bar with control to the ground. Repeat for the desired number of reps.

> **PRO CUE:** Make sure that the middle of the barbell is lined up with the middle of your feet. Line up the knot in your tied shoelaces right in the middle of the bar to approximate this.

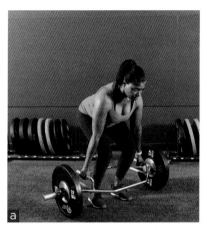
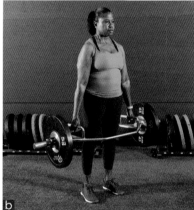

FIGURE 11.11   High hex bar deadlift.

CHAPTER 12

POWER DEVELOPMENT, FINISHERS, AND METABOLIC INTERVALS

Power development is a priority in these programs because as we age, power is one of the first things we lose. Power refers to moving a load as fast as possible. That load could be your body weight jumping or exploding off the ground, or it could be slamming a medicine ball into the floor or a wall.

Metabolic intervals and finishers are the same thing. The difference is that one is done as a short burst at the end of a strength workout (a finisher), and the other is done as a separate metabolic interval training session. Many of the power exercises also double as metabolically demanding exercises that you could use for an interval in your metabolic workout.

BOX JUMP

You've got the power to fly through the air and land on a box! A positive mental attitude is most important during this exercise. If you think you can or think you can't, you're absolutely right!

Position

Stand with your feet shoulder-width apart in front of a sturdy box, starting with one 12 inches tall (figure 12.1a). As you progress, you can increase the height of the box.

Movement

Bend your knees and jump onto the box (figure 12.1b), landing with both feet flat, your hips directly above your knees, your knees bent, and your chest up (figure 12.1c). Step off the box (do not jump) and return to the start position to repeat for the desired number of repetitions.

> PRO CUE: If you cannot land with your hips above your knees, the box height is too high.

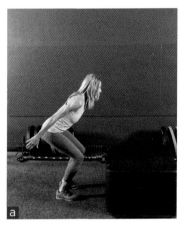 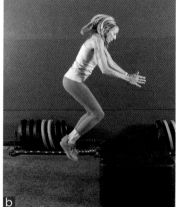 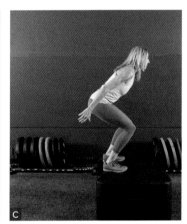

FIGURE 12.1   Box jump.

EXPLOSIVE STEP-UP

This exercise works great as a power exercise, metabolic finisher, or interval for your metabolic workout. During your strength workout, you've been strengthening your legs with step-ups, and this exercise turns that strength into an explosive movement.

Position

Stand facing a step or bench at about knee height with a tall, proud chest and shoulders down. Place one foot on top of the step (figure 12.2a).

Movement

Lean your body weight onto the foot on the step to drive that leg into the step and explosively lift your body into the air (figure 12.2b). Switch legs midair to land with the opposite foot on the step and the other foot on the floor (figure 12.2c), ready to repeat on the opposite leg. As you get stronger, increase the height of the step up to hip height as long as you are still moving quickly and are able to get height into the air.

PRO CUE: Drive your head toward the ceiling with each jump.

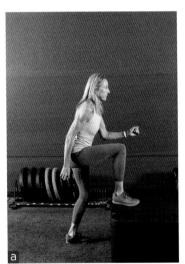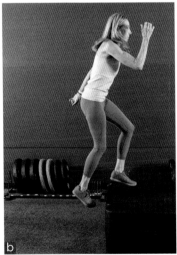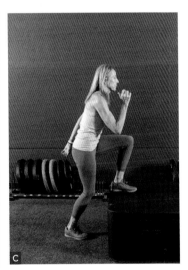

FIGURE 12.2 Explosive step-up.

MEDICINE BALL TALL-KNEELING CHEST THROW

In this exercise, you'll use only your upper body to throw the medicine ball, developing power through your arms, shoulders, and chest. Check that the wall you throw the medicine ball against is solid, such as a cement or block wall. You do not want to throw a weighted ball against drywall because it will go right through. You can also do this as a partner exercise, throwing the ball to each other.

Position

Kneel 4 to 5 feet away from a wall with your knees shoulder-width apart, holding a medicine ball at chest height (figure 12.3*a*). Use a medicine ball that will not bounce back at you too hard.

Movement

Push the ball from your chest as fast as you can, driving the ball toward the wall (figure 12.3*b*), and release it so that the ball hits the wall. The harder you throw, the harder it will rebound. Either catch the ball or let it fall to the ground. Pick up the ball and repeat for the desired number of reps.

> **PRO CUE:** Keep your torso in a vertical plank position during the throw, engaging the abdominals and glutes. Visualize throwing the ball with enough force to attempt to break the ball or break the wall.

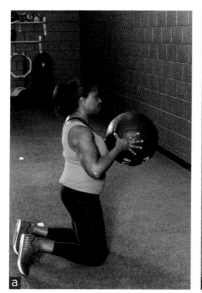 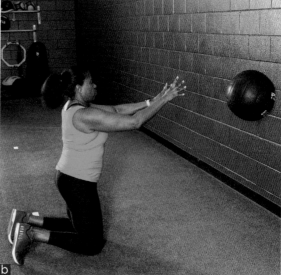

FIGURE 12.3   Medicine ball tall-kneeling chest throw.

MEDICINE BALL CHEST THROW

Medicine ball throws to a wall are one of my favorites. Being able to throw something with everything you've got is gratifying. Check that the wall you throw the medicine ball against is solid, such as a cement or block wall. You do not want to throw a weighted ball against drywall because it will go right through. You can also do this as a partner exercise, throwing the ball to each other.

Position

Stand four to five feet away, facing the wall, with your feet outside of shoulder-width apart as you hold a medicine ball at chest height (figure 12.4a). Use a medicine ball that will not bounce back at you too hard.

Movement

Using your entire body, throw the ball from the chest as fast as you can (figure 12.4b); drive the ball toward the wall and release to have it make an impact on the wall. The harder you throw, the harder it will rebound. Either catch the ball or let it fall to the ground. Pick up the ball and repeat for the desired number of reps. As a metabolic interval option, you can perform the medicine ball chest throw with a forward step to be able to throw harder and with more leverage.

> **PRO CUE:** Visualize throwing the ball with enough force to attempt to break the ball or break the wall.

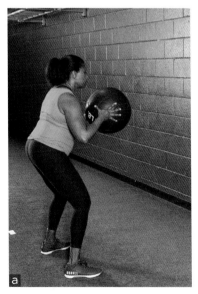
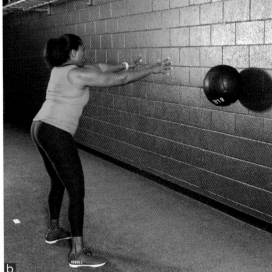

FIGURE 12.4   Medicine ball chest throw.

MEDICINE BALL HALF-KNEELING CHOP THROW

In this exercise, you'll throw the medicine ball in a rotational movement, which is an undertrained yet important movement type. Using your upper body only to throw the medicine ball develops power through your arms, shoulders, and chest, along with putting your core to work. Check that the wall you throw the medicine ball against is solid, such as a cement or block wall. You do not want to throw a weighted ball against drywall because it will go right through. You can also do this as a partner exercise, throwing the ball to each other.

Position

Kneel sideways about four to five feet away from the wall, with your outside foot on the floor to create a 90-degree angle with your leg and your inside knee (the one closest to the wall) on the floor stacked under your hip (figure 12.5*a*). Hold a medicine ball.

Movement

Raise the medicine ball up and away from the wall, extending your upper body as far as you can to create tension to throw (figure 12.5*b*). As hard and as fast as you can, drive the ball into the ground in the direction of the wall so that it bounces and then hits the wall (figure 12.5*c*). The harder you throw, the harder the ball will rebound. Either catch the ball when it returns to you or let it fall to the ground. Pick up the ball and repeat for the desired number of reps. Switch to the other side.

> **PRO CUE:** Reach the crown of your head toward the ceiling and keep it there during the performance of the movement.

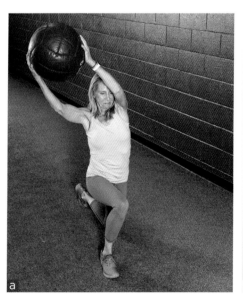 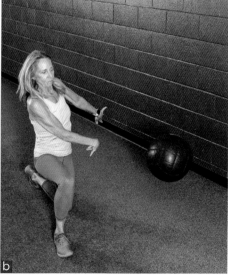

FIGURE 12.5 Medicine ball half-kneeling chop throw.

MEDICINE BALL SIDE THROW

Rotational movements are often forgotten in exercise programs, but they are oh so important. With this rotational move, you'll be throwing a medicine ball using the power of your entire body as you rotate from the hips. Check that the wall you throw the medicine ball against is solid, such as a cement or block wall. You do not want to throw a weighted ball against drywall because it will go right through. You can also do this as a partner exercise, throwing the ball to each other.

Position

Stand sideways to the wall, about four to five feet away, with your feet outside of shoulder-width apart as you hold a medicine ball in front of you with your arms straight (figure 12.6*a*). Use a medicine ball that will not bounce back at you too hard.

Movement

With your feet planted, rotate your body away from the wall as you take the medicine ball as far away from it as possible (figure 12.6*b*). Wind up, then snap your hips through to turn back toward the wall (figure 12.6*c*) and release the ball to make an impact on the wall. The harder you throw, the harder the ball will rebound. Either catch the ball or let it fall to the ground. Pick up the ball and repeat for the desired number of reps. Switch to the other side.

> **PRO CUE:** Throw the ball with power from your hips, snapping them through to create the power. Visualize throwing the ball with enough force to attempt to break the ball or break the wall.

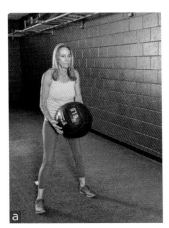 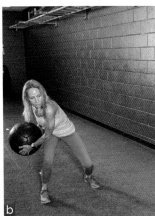 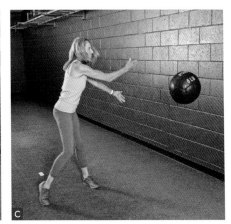

FIGURE 12.6   Medicine ball side throw.

MEDICINE BALL FLOOR SLAM

Be sure that the floor you are slamming the medicine ball to doesn't have people living underneath; it'll be pretty loud if you're doing this right!

Position

Stand with your feet shoulder-width apart, holding a medicine ball at chest height. Use a medicine ball that does not bounce back at you. If the ball does bounce back, be careful to dodge the rebound after you throw the ball.

Movement

Raise the medicine ball overhead as you extend onto your toes, extending your hips and shoulders to create as much tension as you can (figure 12.7a). Use your entire body to slam the ball into the floor (figure 12.7b). Pick up the ball and repeat for the desired number of reps.

> **PRO CUE:** Set the body in a vertical plank at the top of the motion; engage the abdominals and glutes. Imagine that you are trying to crack the ball open on the floor when you slam it down.

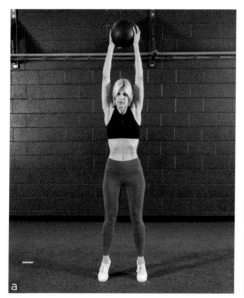 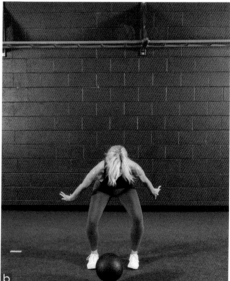

FIGURE 12.7   Medicine ball floor slam.

SANDBAG CLEAN

Once you have progressed and improved your power development, it's time to add some Olympic lifting movements. These are some of the most effective power development exercises available. The Olympic movements include a clean (which is what you'll be doing in this exercise), a snatch (an advanced exercise in which you move the weight from the ground to overhead), and a push press (which can be done following a clean). In this exercise, you will use a sandbag to learn how to do a clean.

Position

Stand with your feet outside shoulder-width apart and a sandbag lying across your feet (figure 12.8a). Start with the lightest sandbag and progress to a heavier bag.

Movement

Bend down and grab the handles on the bag; think about pulling them apart to engage your lats (figure 12.8b). In one fast movement, explode up, bringing the bag up along your legs to land on the front of your arms in a front carry position (figure 12.8c). Stand tall at the top of the movement. Return the bag to the ground and repeat for the desired number of reps.

> **PRO CUE:** Keep the bag very close the body on the way up and the way down, as if zipping and unzipping a jacket. The hips provide the primary drive for this exercise; the arms serve as guides.

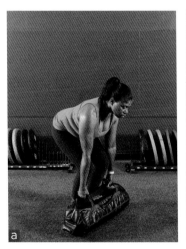 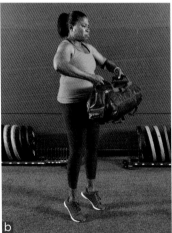 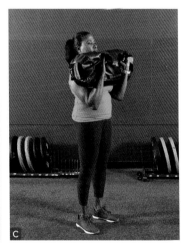

FIGURE 12.8   Sandbag clean.

SANDBAG CLEAN AND PRESS

Easier to learn than a kettlebell clean, this exercise could be your first step to mastering the Olympic lift called the clean. Because it's softer than a kettlebell or barbell, the sandbag is an excellent learning tool. Once you clean the sandbag, you'll press it overhead.

Position

Stand with your feet outside of shoulder-width with a sandbag placed across the tops of your feet. Reach down to grab the handles of the sandbag as you reach your hips back (figure 12.9a), maintaining a flat, neutral spine and engaging the posterior chain so you are ready to explode and lift the sandbag to the rack position.

Movement

Drive your feet into the ground using your lower body as you powerfully straighten your legs. Explode the sandbag up, keeping your elbows high as it flies up, then tuck your elbows underneath the sandbag to catch it in the rack position (figure 12.9b and c). Then bend your knees as if to jump and power the bag to land overhead with your arms straight next to your ears. Lower the sandbag under control back to the rack position, then the start position. Repeat quickly for the work period while maintaining form.

> **PRO CUE:** Your arms are like ropes simply holding the load that your legs and hips are powering into the air. As you drive it overhead, use your hips and legs to create the force.

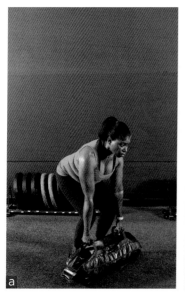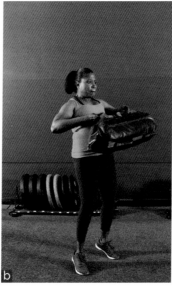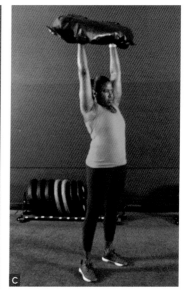

FIGURE 12.9   Sandbag clean and press.

ALTERNATING KETTLEBELL CLEAN

If you've never been coached on a kettlebell clean, I suggest that you ask a kettlebell coach at your gym to give you a few pointers.

Position

Stand with your feet outside of shoulder-width, with a kettlebell placed between your heels. Reach down to grab the handle of the kettlebell with one arm as you reach your hips back (figure 12.10a). Maintain a flat, neutral spine. Engage the posterior chain so you are ready to explode the kettlebell up to the rack position.

Movement

Drive your feet into the ground and use your lower body as you powerfully straighten your legs and explode the kettlebell up. Keep your elbow high as the kettlebell flies up, then tuck your elbow underneath it to catch it in the rack position (figure 12.10b). Lower the kettlebell with control back to the start position and switch arms (figure 12.10c), lifting the kettlebell with the opposite arm (figure 12.10d). Alternate for the desired number of reps or, if working for a certain time, move as fast as you can while maintaining your form.

Until you learn the movement, you can perform a "cheat" clean. Use both hands to lift the kettlebell with more control, using your second hand to spot the kettlebell.

> **PRO CUE:** Think *smooth* with this one; as you pop the kettlebell up, drive your arm through smoothly to have the kettlebell land on your wrist so that it doesn't cause bruising. You may want to wear wristbands to protect your wrists as you're learning the form.

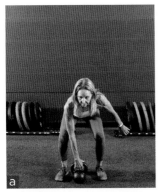
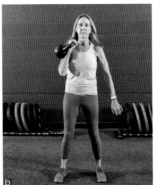
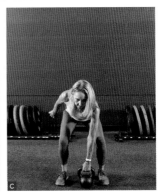

FIGURE 12.10 Alternating kettlebell clean.

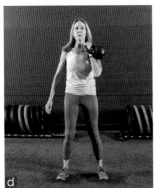

KETTLEBELL SWING

If you've never been coached on a kettlebell swing, I suggest you ask a kettlebell coach at your gym to give you some pointers. This is a fantastic exercise but can take some coaching to get it right.

Position

Stand with your feet outside of shoulder width, facing a kettlebell about a foot in front of you. Grab the handle of the kettlebell with both hands as you reach your hips back, maintaining a flat, neutral spine and engaging the posterior chain (figure 12.11a).

Movement

Pick up the kettlebell and hike it between your legs (figure 12.11b); imagine you are going to throw it toward the wall behind you (but don't let go!). Keep your chest proud and your feet planted on the floor as you hinge from the hips. As the kettlebell swings back, use your hips to brake the kettlebell while switching the momentum to swing forward in front of you. Allow the kettlebell to travel up to chest height with your arms straight (figure 12.11c). Your legs are straight, and your body is in a vertical plank position before you let the kettlebell swing back through your legs as you hinge your hips. Repeat for the desired number of reps.

> **PRO CUE:** Think "Snap!" as you snap your hips through to power that kettlebell up!

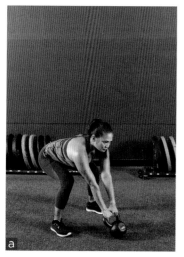 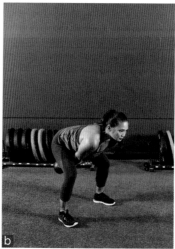 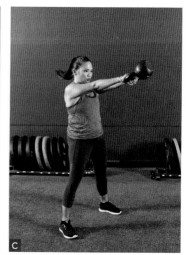

FIGURE 12.11 Kettlebell swing.

BODYWEIGHT SQUAT

Most likely you have performed many bodyweight squats in your lifetime. In fact, sitting on a chair and standing back up is a version of a bodyweight squat. It's one of the most frequently used functional movements, and now you'll perform it as fast as you can with good form to get your heart rate cranking for a metabolic interval.

Position

Stand with your feet shoulder-width apart and your hands behind your head or straight out in front of you, your posture tall (figure 12.12a).

Movement

Bend your knees and hinge at the hips as you lower into a squat until your thighs are at or below parallel to the floor (figure 12.12b). Push through your feet as you return to standing. Keep your knees tracking over your toes and your heels on the floor the entire time. Repeat for the desired number of reps.

> **PRO CUE:** Posture up! Show off that logo on your T-shirt!

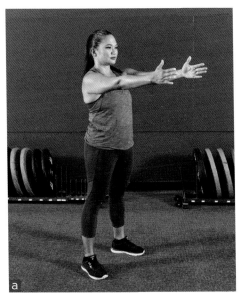 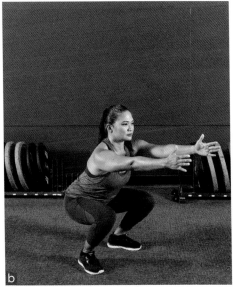

FIGURE 12.12   Bodyweight squat.

SANDBAG BEAR HUG SQUAT

Adding in an upper-body squeeze with load to the bodyweight squat makes you work harder in this exercise.

Position

Stand with your feet shoulder-width apart, holding a sandbag in front of you perpendicular to your body. Wrap your arms around the sandbag, pulling it toward your chest and holding it like a baby while keeping your back muscles engaged and your chest lifted (figure 12.13a).

Movement

Holding the sandbag firmly to engage your upper back and arms, bend your knees and hinge at the hips to lower yourself into a squat until your thighs are at or below parallel to the floor (figure 12.13b). Return to the starting position and repeat for the desired number of reps. Keep your knees tracking over your toes and your heels on the floor the entire time.

> **PRO CUE:** Dip into that squat, then drive up strong. Dip and drive!

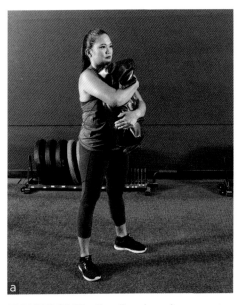 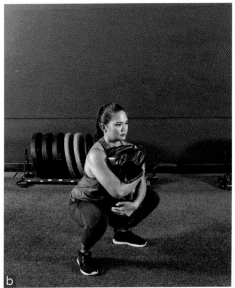

FIGURE 12.13 Sandbag bear hug squat.

JUMP SQUAT

Taking the bodyweight squat up a notch and using your power to drive yourself off the ground in a jump squat is one way to really get your heart rate up quick.

Position

Stand with your feet shoulder-width apart and your hands behind your head, your elbows out and your posture tall.

Movement

Bend your knees and hinge at the hips as you lower into a squat until the tops of your thighs are at or below parallel to the floor (figure 12.14*a*). Next, rapidly drive out of the bottom of the squat and propel yourself into the air (figure 12.14*b*). Land softly and quietly and return to the bottom of the squat position for the next repetition as soon as your feet land. Repeat for the desired number of reps.

> **PRO CUE:** Jump as high as you can, powering yourself off the floor. Keep your knees pushed out and your heels on the floor as you lower into the squat.

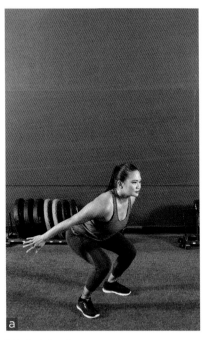 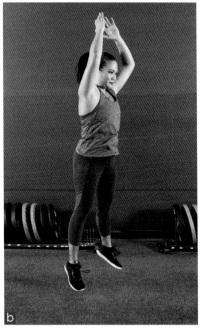

FIGURE 12.14   Jump squat.

BURPEE, SQUAT THRUST, OR MEDICINE BALL SQUAT THRUST

The standard burpee is a staple in metabolic interval workouts because it works so well to get your heart rate up, engages your whole body, and is a challenging exercise to perform. Be careful not to get sloppy with your form; you can regress the exercise as needed, until you're ready to progress. The difference between a squat thrust and a burpee is whether you jump off the ground. You can choose which version you need to do to get your heart rate pumping. Putting your hands on a medicine ball decreases the range of motion, creating an easier version of the squat thrust.

Position

Stand with your feet together and your arms at your sides. If you're using a medicine ball, set the ball in front of you.

Movement

Bend down and touch the floor with your hands (figure 12.15*a*). Put your weight on your hands and jump your legs behind you so that you are extended into a plank position. Do not let your back sag (figure 12.15*b*). Jump your feet back to your hands again and stand up (squat thrust) or jump into the air (burpee). Repeat for the desired number of reps.

To regress this exercise, place your hands on a medicine ball (figure 12.15*c*), box, or bench rather than the floor. You can also step one foot back at a time instead of jumping both feet back at the same time.

> **PRO CUE:** Find the version of this exercise you can do properly because it's often done with poor form.

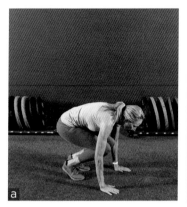 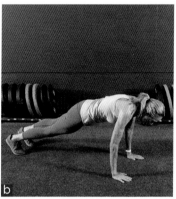 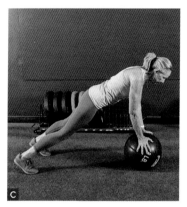

FIGURE 12.15   Burpee, squat thrust, or medicine ball squat thrust.

WALKING LUNGE

This variation turns the lunge into a locomotion metabolic exercise. Alternating the legs as you walk forward so that neither side stays under tension gets your heart rate pumping.

Position

Make sure you have enough space to take at least 10 lunges forward before turning around. Stand tall with a proud posture, your eyes on the horizon and your arms on your hips or behind your head.

Movement

Take a big step forward with one leg and lower into a full range-of-motion lunge, keeping your front heel down as your back knee grazes the floor behind you (figure 12.16a). Keep your eyes on the horizon with a proud posture, your shoulders down and back. Drive into the ground with the front leg, pushing yourself back up to standing as your rear leg comes off the ground to come through and step forward to perform the next lunge (figure 12.16b). Repeat, alternating sides and moving forward for the desired number of reps.

PRO CUE: Imagine gluing the heel of the front leg to the ground as you pull yourself through to the next lunge.

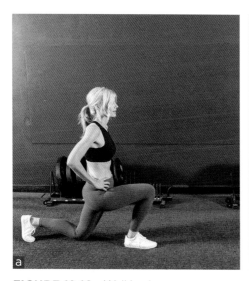 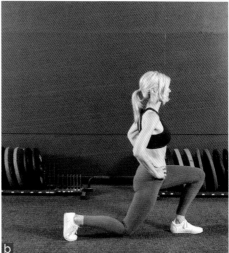

FIGURE 12.16 Walking lunge.

LUNGE WITH ROTATION

Adding a torso rotation to alternating lunges increases the demand on your body, adding one more plane of motion to work your balance and ability to stabilize.

Position

Stand with your feet shoulder-width apart and your arms at your sides.

Movement

Step forward with your right leg into a deep lunge (figure 12.17a), keeping your front heel down as your left knee grazes the floor behind you. At the bottom of the lunge, rotate your torso to the right to increase the stretch in the left hip flexor (figure 12.17b). Drive through the right heel and return to the start position. Repeat on the left leg. Alternate legs as fast as you can while maintaining your form for the amount of time.

> PRO CUE: Imagine gluing the heel of the front leg to the ground, engaging your hip and keeping your knee tracking over your second toe as you drive through your lunges.

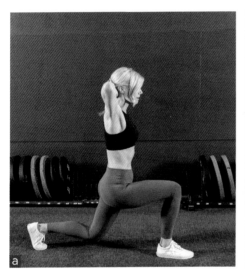 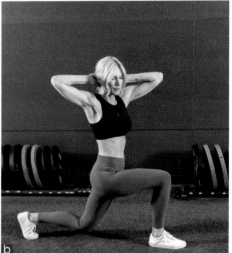

FIGURE 12.17 Lunge with rotation.

LUNGE JUMP

Adding a jump to alternating lunges creates one of the hardest exercises you'll do. This is an advanced exercise. Start with alternating lunges without a jump before progressing to lunge jumps.

Position

Stand with your feet together, then step one foot back about 12 to 18 inches, keeping your legs straight.

Movement

Bend both knees to lower yourself into the bottom of a lunge (figure 12.18a), and then explosively launch yourself into the air, switching the position of the legs in midair (figure 12.18b). On landing (your feet with be opposite of where they were at the start; figure 12.18c), lower into another lunge and repeat the explosive jumps for the desired number of reps or time.

> **PRO CUE:** Maintain a tall posture and keep moving as you explode up.

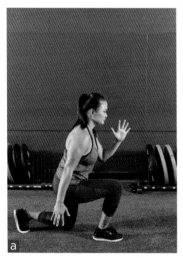
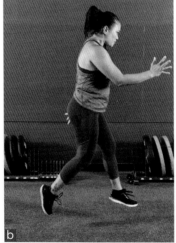
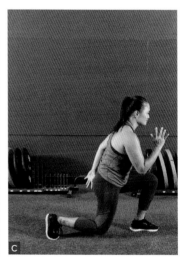

FIGURE 12.18   Lunge jump.

SANDBAG DYNAMIC REVERSE LUNGE

By getting dynamic with the lunge pattern, this exercise actively stretches the hip flexors while firing up the lower body.

Position

Stand with your feet hip-width apart and hold a sandbag in a front-loaded position against your chest. Keep a tall posture and proud chest with your shoulders down and back.

Movement

Shift your weight to one side as you step one leg behind you and lower into a lunge. Do not narrow your stance, or it will make it more difficult to balance. Lower until the back knee almost touches the floor. Brace your abs to keep the pelvis stable as you lunge. Push through the front foot to return to the start position. Alternate sides for the number of reps.

PRO CUE: Think about pulling the sandbag into your chest to engage your upper back with a tall posture.

SANDBAG DYNAMIC REVERSE LUNGE WITH ROTATION

Adding a rotation while holding a sandbag in front of your body, letting the sandbag swing with the rotation, really fires up your muscles to work harder from your core to your legs to your hips.

Position

Stand with your feet hip-width apart, holding a sandbag with both hands hanging in front of your body at the middle of your thigh. Keep a tall posture and a proud chest with your shoulders down and back.

Movement

Shift your weight to one side as you step one leg behind you and lower into a lunge. Do not narrow your stance, or it will make it more difficult to balance. Lower until the back knee almost touches the floor as you rotate your upper body to the opposite direction as the leg stepping back, letting the sandbag fall to the outside the lunged leg. Brace your abs to keep the pelvis stable, stabilizing your torso as you lunge while keeping your front foot cemented to the ground. Push through the front foot to return to the start position. Alternate sides for the number of reps.

PRO CUE: As the sandbag drops to the side, resist the load pulling you in that direction.

ALTERNATING LATERAL LUNGE

Time to work side to side in the frontal plane. Movement in this plane is often neglected, because many workout programs include only sagittal (front to back) exercises. It is important to work your body in all three planes of motion.

Position

Stand with your feet shoulder-width apart and your arms at your sides.

Movement

Step out with your right leg into a wide stance. Bend your right leg as you lower into a side lunge while keeping your left leg straight (figure 12.19a). Go as deep as you can go while keeping your right heel on the floor. Try to get full range of motion and then push off the right leg and return to the start position. Repeat to your left side (figure 12.19b). Alternate back and forth. You can add a hop in between each lunge as you move from one side to the other or hold a sandbag if you want to make the exercise harder.

PRO CUE: Think of this as a touch-and-go movement, driving off your outside leg quickly to move to the other side.

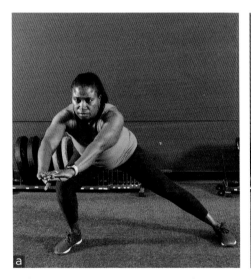 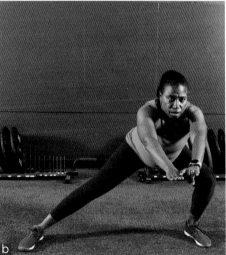

FIGURE 12.19   Alternating lateral lunge.

LADDER DRILLS

A floor ladder is a fun addition to your workouts, plus a way to test your agility and raise your heart rate. You may see ladders used on fields during athlete training, but most functional training gyms also have ladders. If you don't have a ladder, you can pretend there are lines on the floor.

Position

Place the floor ladder in a space away from where people walk or work out. Start each drill by standing at one end of the ladder.

Movement

Choose from any of the patterns that follow.

Forward Two In/Two Out

You may feel like you're doing the cha-cha in this simple drill. Be sure to move those feet as fast as you can! Moving your feet as quickly as possible, step two feet into the first square of the ladder and then one foot outside the ladder on each side, to straddle the ladder (figure 12.20). Step back into the next square with both feet and then straddle the ladder with each foot. Continue down the entire length of the ladder, moving as fast as you can for the allotted work time. If you get to the end, turn around and come back until time is up.

> **PRO CUE:** When first performing this movement, it helpful to think "in-in, out-out." Add speed as you learn the pattern.

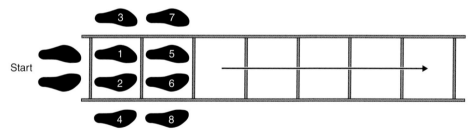

FIGURE 12.20   Forward two in/two out ladder drill.

Hopscotch

Remember hopscotch? This one will take you back to your childhood! Hop on one foot in the first square, then hop both feet outside of the next square to straddle the ladder (figure 12.21). Hop on the other foot into the third square and straddle the fourth square. Continue hopscotching forward to the end of the ladder for the allotted time. If you get to the end, turn around and come back until time is up.

PRO CUE: Move like the ground is hot, thinking "Hop and go!"

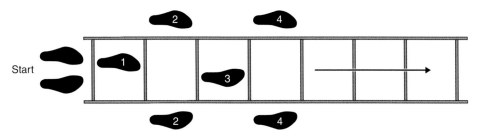

FIGURE 12.21 Hopscotch ladder drill.

Ickey Shuffle

The Ickey Shuffle is named after Elbert "Ickey" Woods' touchdown dance. It's been adopted as an agility ladder drill for athletes and will get you moving fast with rapid feet and overall speed. Step one foot and then the other into the first square. Then step outside of the ladder with the foot you started with as you lift the trailing leg (figure 12.22)—right (inside square), left (inside square), then right step outside. The trailing leg then becomes the lead leg as you step into the next square—left (inside square), right (inside square), then left step outside. Continue for the allotted time. If you get to the end, turn around and come back until time is up.

PRO CUE: Start slowly as you say out loud, "1,2, out, 1,2, out" until you get the rhythm, then pick up the speed.

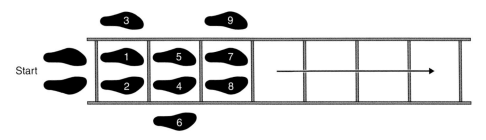

FIGURE 12.22 Ickey shuffle ladder drill.

Two Steps/One Step

In this drill, you will stay in the ladder squares the entire time, moving quickly through them. Be sure to move those feet as fast as you can! Moving your feet as quickly as possible, step two feet into the first square of the ladder, then one foot into the next square (figure 12.23). Two feet go into the next square, and then one foot into the next, alternating the lead foot each time. Continue down the entire length of the ladder, moving as fast as you can for the allotted work time. If you get to the end, turn around and come back until time is up.

> **PRO CUE:** Talk yourself through the drill as you're learning it, "1, 2, 1 and 2, 1, 2" and so on, then pick up the speed.

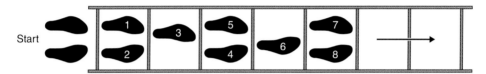

FIGURE 12.23   Two steps/one step ladder drill.

Lateral Shuffle

You'll take your ladder drill sideways this time. Be sure to move those feet as fast as you can! Stand with one side to the ladder. Moving your feet as quickly as possible, step one foot and then the other into the first square of the ladder (figure 12.24). Step one foot and then the other outside the ladder, moving sideways up the ladder. Continue moving sideways up the ladder, placing one foot and then the other in the next square and then one foot and the other back out. Continue down the entire length of the ladder, moving as fast as you can for the allotted work time. If you get to the end, turn around and come back until time is up. If you are performing the drill more than once, begin the next set with your other side to the ladder.

> **PRO CUE:** Start slowly to get your coordination, saying, "In, in, out, out" until you have it, then pick up the speed.

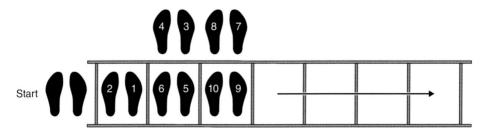

FIGURE 12.24   Lateral shuffle ladder drill.

JUMP ROPE

Jumping rope is an oldie but a goodie. You have lots of options for variations in how you jump, and if you don't have a jump rope, you can pretend that you're jumping over a rope.

Position

Stand with your feet together and hold the handles of the jump rope loosely in each hand, with the rope behind your feet.

Movement

Swing the jump rope up and over your head. As it passes under your feet, either jump over with both feet (figure 12.25a) or hop on one foot at a time (figure 12.25b). Start slowly with a small jump in between each pass of the rope under your feet if needed. As you practice, work on turning the rope faster until you are jumping over it quickly. If you trip on the rope, it's no problem; just start again.

PRO CUE: Stay light and springy on your feet, adding that double hop as you get started.

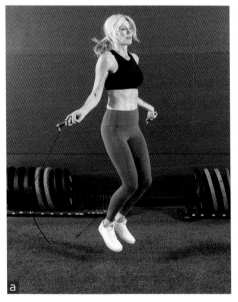 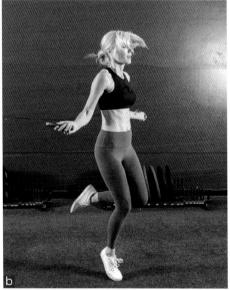

FIGURE 12.25 Jump rope, with (a) both feet and (b) hopping on one foot at a time.

BATTLE ROPE INTERVALS

Battle ropes came on the fitness scene around 2006, and now most functional training gyms have at least one set of battle ropes. If you don't have access to them, perform bodyweight squats or squat jumps instead. Using the battle ropes, you'll be able to elevate your heart rate while using your entire body, which is the goal of a finisher. You'll make movements with your upper body while creating power with your lower body.

Position

Anchor the middle of the battle rope to a sturdy object. Stand with your feet shoulder-width apart, facing the anchor point and holding one end of the rope in each hand. Bend the knees to lower into a partial squat and brace the core.

Movement

Choose from any of the following patterns. You can switch up the motion every 10 seconds or stay with one pattern the entire 30 seconds.

> **PRO CUE:** Stay in an athletic position while performing each pattern. Send waves of energy to the anchor point, using fast, whipping actions. You don't want to use slow, labored motions.

Drumroll

Alternate lifting each arm up and down, as if you're drumming (figure 12.26), sending a snake motion down both ropes as you bend your legs while moving the hips and torso to get a rhythm of movement. Perform this movement as quickly as possible while getting the entire rope moving. You can progress this to walk toward the anchor point and back while continuing the drumroll.

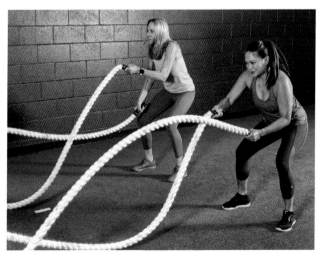

FIGURE 12.26   Drumroll battle rope drill.

Giddyup

Make a big upward movement with both arms and then slam the rope to the floor as if telling a horse to giddyup (figure 12.27). Repeat. Each time, use your lower body by lifting onto your toes on the up motion and lower into a squat on the down motion. Perform this movement as quickly as possible while getting the entire rope moving. You can progress this by adding in a jump squat as you lift the arms and rope into the air.

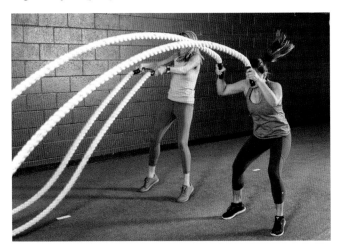

FIGURE 12.27   Giddyup battle rope drill.

Outward Circles

Move both arms up and out, then down and in, to make a circle motion with each arm (figure 12.28). Bend your legs up and down to get momentum, repeating the circles as you are moving the entire rope in this circle motion as quickly as possible.

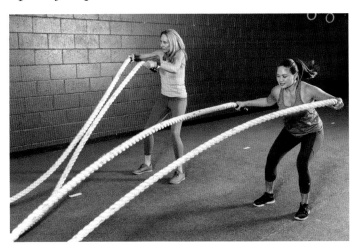

FIGURE 12.28   Outward circles battle rope drill.

Side to Side

Holding both ropes with the ends pointing up, step to one side while bringing both ropes up and over to one hip (figure 12.29). Return to the start, then step to the other side, bringing both ropes up and over to that hip. Continue back and forth, moving the rope side to side as quickly as possible.

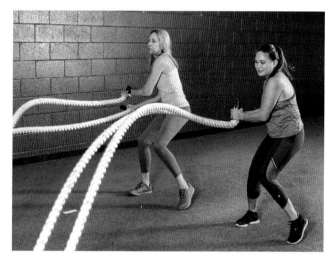

FIGURE 12.29 Side to side battle rope drill.

FAN BIKE SPRINT

Fan bikes, sometimes called air or assault bikes, have handles that you pump with the upper body while you pedal with your lower body. They are the ultimate way to get your heart rate cranking during a metabolic interval and work great for intense interval training. The fan inside the front wheel provides air resistance for upright bikes with arm handles, so you can use both your legs and arms to propel the air. You can also do these sprint intervals on a spin bike if you don't have access to a fan bike. As with all finishers, the goal is to get the heart rate up, challenging yourself aerobically at the end of your workout.

Position

Before getting on the bike, stand next to it to adjust the seat height to the same height as your hips. When you're seated on the bike, you should be able to easily reach the pedals when your legs are fully extended at the bottom position (figure 12.30).

Movement

Use your legs to pedal and your arms to push the handles, alternating back and forth as hard as you can continuously for the work interval. Take note of the number on the power meter and aim to match or beat it on your next interval.

> PRO CUE: Make the fan as loud as possible during the sprint. This is one way to gauge that your effort is high!

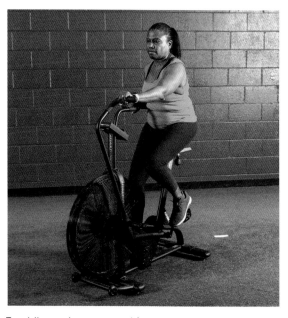

FIGURE 12.30   Fan bike sprint start position.

TREADMILL SPRINT OR FLOOR SPRINT

Sprints are always a great choice to get your heart rate up, burn some calories, and improve your fitness. We have a Woodway self-propelled treadmill that works great when you jump on and sprint. You can also use a regular treadmill, but it may take a little more time to bump up the speed each time you get on, or use a 20-meter (22 yd) space in a group fitness room of your gym to hit some sprints.

Position

Stand tall, rising onto the balls of your feet, feeling light and fast and ready to go.

Movement

Either as you increase your speed on the treadmill or as you step forward to sprint across the gym, think about pulling the floor behind you with each step as you propel yourself forward. Your body will be at a slight forward lean. Your arms are bent at your sides, pumping back and forth; your eyes are on the horizon; and your shoulders are relaxed.

> **PRO CUE:** Keep your eyes on the horizon and pump those arms.

STAIR CLIMBER

Find some stairs to run up and down or use a stair climber machine to push your heart rate up fast to get an interval training response. There's nothing like climbing stairs to get your heart rate pumping!

Position

Face the stairs or stair climber, ready to start climbing. If you're using a stair climber, you'll need to crank up the speed as you get moving.

Movement

Place your entire foot on the first step and drive through the step to lift your body. Bring your trailing leg through to place it on the next step, alternating your feet as you climb the stairs. Increase the speed to really get your heart rate pumping to a pace you can safely keep up with while keeping your eyes on the horizon with a proud posture, your shoulders down and back. If you're on a stair climber and need to hold on to the guard rails, grasp them lightly; do not lean your body weight onto the guard rails.

> **PRO CUE:** Posture up! Keep the chest up, eyes up, and hands off the rails!

MOUNTAIN CLIMBER

Mountain climbers are a great full-body metabolic exercise that boosts your heart rate. It can be done as a beginner or an extremely advanced progression. The core strength you've been building in your strength workouts will come in handy for this one.

Position

Begin on the floor in a plank position with your body weight supported on your hands and toes (figure 12.31*a*). Grip the floor with your palms and ensure your head, shoulders, upper back, and hips are in alignment. If you look down and see your abdomen pooching like a tent, think about drawing it up and in to engage the deep muscles of your abdominals without lifting your hips.

Movement

Without moving from your hips to your head, lift one foot off the ground as you drive that knee under you and up toward your chest without rounding your back (figure 12.31*b*). The opposite leg is locked straight. Return the first leg to the start position and switch legs as you bring the opposite knee up toward your chest. Pick up the pace to drive one knee, then the other toward your chest as fast as you can while maintaining your body position. Grip the floor with your hands and keep your shoulders down and back. You can make this exercise easier by doing it on an incline with your hands on a box or bench. You can make this exercise harder by placing your feet on an unstable surface such as a TRX or slider discs.

> **PRO CUE:** Think "drive, drive" with those knees, alternating quickly while keeping your hips level.

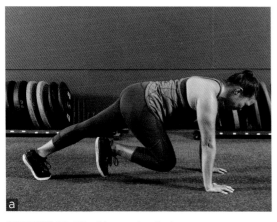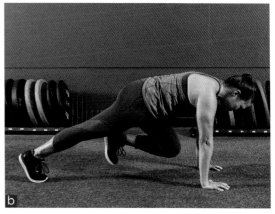

FIGURE 12.31 Mountain climber.

PRONE CROSS TOE TOUCH

This exercise takes a bit of coordination as you touch your foot to your hand, keeping the rest of your body still while moving the legs.

Position

Begin on the floor in a plank position with your body weight supported on your hands and toes (figure 12.32*a*).

Movement

Cross your right leg under your body and touch your foot to your left hand (figure 12.32*b*), then return the right foot to the starting position. Next, cross your left foot under your body to touch your right hand, and return. Keep the torso from moving too much, with most of the movement bending at the hip. Continue to alternate legs.

PRO CUE: Stay low. Think about moving from your core.

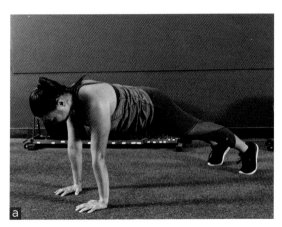 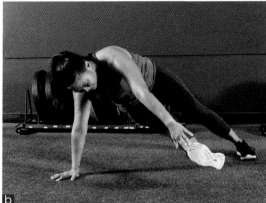

FIGURE 12.32 Prone cross toe touch.

SPIDERMAN

This exercise helps you work on flexibility while elevating your heart rate. It's a dynamic exercise that can be regressed if needed as you learn the movement.

Position

Begin in a plank position with your body weight supported on your hands and toes. Grip the floor with your palms and keep your head, shoulders, upper back, and hips in alignment. If you look down and see your abdomen pooching like a tent, think about drawing it up and in to engage the deep muscles of your abdominals without lifting your hips.

Movement

Explode off the floor and land with your left hand reaching out past your head in front of you, your left leg straight back, and your right hand and foot underneath you and next to each other on the floor, as if you were Spider-Man climbing a wall (figure 12.33*a*). Explode and switch your arms and legs in midair so that the right arm reaches in front of you, the right leg is back, and the left hand and left foot meet underneath you (figure 12.33*b*). Continue to alternate.

If this version is too advanced, you can make the exercise easier by bringing one foot to the outside of your hand on the same side in line with the shoulder while keeping your body as still as possible from your hips to your head. The opposite leg is straight as you keep your body in one straight line. Return that foot to the start position and switch to bring the opposite foot up to the outside of the hand. Alternate back and forth as quickly as you can while keeping your body in a plank position. An even easier version is to place your hands on a step or bench and bring each foot forward to be in line with your same-side knee or hip instead of the shoulder.

> **PRO CUE:** The ground is hot, so move as quickly as you can, exploding into position.

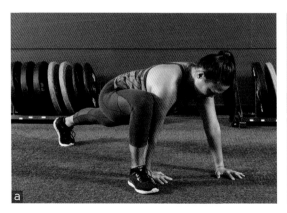 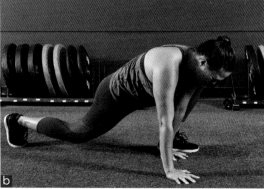

FIGURE 12.33   Spiderman.

FORWARD CRAWL WITH SANDBAG DRAG

Forward crawls seem like such a simple exercise but are one of the hardest exercises you'll do because so many muscles are involved. Add a sandbag into the mix, and your heart rate will be racing as you sweat toward the finish.

Position

Make sure you have space in front of you to crawl across. Place a sandbag on the floor. Position yourself over the sandbag on your hands and knees, then lift your knees off the floor so your full weight is supported on your hands and toes (figure 12.34a). Grip the floor with your palms and ensure your head, shoulders, upper back, and hips are in alignment.

Movement

Grab the handle at the top of the bag with one hand and pull it forward and out from under you (figure 12.34b). Crawl on your hands and feet while maintaining your head, shoulder, and hip alignment until you are positioned over the bag again. Use the opposite hand to pull the bag forward, then crawl forward until you are over the bag. Repeat for the desired amount of time. If you run out of room, turn around and crawl back to where you started.

PRO CUE: Keep the hips low and core engaged.

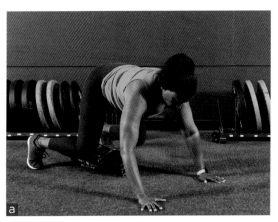 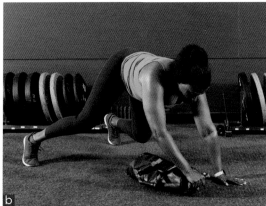

FIGURE 12.34   Forward crawl with sandbag drag.

PART IV

THE AGE STRONG PROGRAM

CHAPTER 13

PROGRAM PRINCIPLES

You understand the importance of strength training as a priority beyond your 40s, have set some powerful goals, and are ready to hit the gym to get started building muscle, improving your movement, and feeling fit, no matter your age. The programs in this book have been designed to progress over each phase following the scientific principles laid out in this chapter and have been used for years with real women over age 40. They've experienced life-changing results; you've been introduced to some of them throughout the book. I also have tested these programs on myself, and hundreds of women at Results Fitness have followed them over the 23 years we've been open. In fact, while writing this book, I'm taking eight women through this exact program as a focus group, inspiring everything you're reading.

This training program is 16 to 20 weeks long. It's broken into four phases, each with a different focus. You'll start with the base phase and then move through each remaining phase of the program. These are the phases:

• *Base phase.* You will begin this program by laying a foundation. The exercises in the base phase address common imbalances and will teach you basic movements such as the squat, lunge, bend, push, pull, and twist so you can execute them properly. This phase will set you up for long-term success, keeping you injury-free, fit, strong, and healthy as you age. During the final week of the base phase, you'll perform a "plus" set to see if your loading was challenging enough. If not, you know to push yourself a bit more in the next phase.

• *Build phase.* Once you've awakened all the right muscles and are moving properly, you're ready for a lower-rep phase. In this phase, you will add load to the movements as you progress, bumping up the intensity. The plus phase at the end will really push you to lift as heavy as you safely can to get the anabolic age-reversing effect we're looking for.

• *Stronger phase.* Continuing to improve your movement, you'll be ready to build volume by increasing the number of reps and the load along with progressing some of the exercises as you get stronger. You'll again finish with a "plus" set during the final week as you learn to properly load each exercise. You should be able to load pretty heavy by the end of this phase, and doing this check will let you know if you're on target.

• *Age strong phase.* In the final phase, you'll hit some baseline strength standards to see if you can perform certain exercises such as a push-up or lift a specific amount of weight, finishing this program stronger than when you started. By hitting these baseline standards (see sidebar), you'll know you are where you need to be to age strong.

Each phase has two or three strength training days per week alternated on nonconsecutive days. These are all total-body workouts, so you will need a day off between each workout to let your body repair and recover.

Part of my philosophy on getting the best results from a fitness program is to train with a purpose or goal in mind. These programs provide a specific focus to keep you from just winging it or going through the motions. The goal is to age strong. Your time in the gym will be used to move you forward to feeling fit, strong, and healthy as you age. By following these programs, you'll know you're doing exactly what you need to do. Every exercise, set, rep, tempo, and rest period will be laid out for you to ensure that you are not wasting your time and can achieve the best results possible.

It is important to understand the scientific principles underlying these workouts and the thought process behind designing them to be able to continue your journey as you age strong. Let's explore each principle in detail.

Baseline Standards

Table 13.1 shows the baseline standards of strength for you to shoot for throughout this program. Calculate your numbers to have a goal in mind as you work through the program, and check them off as you hit them!

TABLE 13.1 **Strength Standards**

Exercise	Reps or time	Load	Your goal
Hollow hold	60 sec	Body weight	Body weight
Push-up	5 reps	Body weight	Body weight
Dumbbell incline bench press	5 reps	25% of body weight	
Goblet split squat	5 reps	25% of body weight	
Dumbbell two-point row	5 reps	25% of body weight	
Front plank	60 sec	Body weight	Body weight
Side plank	30 sec	Body weight	Body weight
Kettlebell deadlift	5 reps	75% of body weight	
Dumbbell one-leg RDL	5 reps	40% of body weight	
Front squat	5 reps	50% of body weight	
High hex bar deadlift	5 reps	75% body weight	
Stationary split squat (two free weights)	5 reps	20% body weight total (so two 15-lb [7 kg] dumbbells would equal 30 lb [14 kg] and be 20% body weight for a 150 lb [68 kg] female)	

PRINCIPLE 1: STRENGTH FIRST

As you age, it's crucial that strength training becomes the first priority of your fitness training. If you don't actively do something to combat aging, you'll gradually lose muscle every year through a process known as sarcopenia. The awesome thing is that you can reverse that! In chapter 1, I went deep into the science of losing muscle, so if you need convincing, go back and reread that chapter. The benefits of lifting weights far outweigh any other type of exercise.

Usually, women prioritize aerobic workouts such as walking or running and lift weights only if they have extra time. As we age, the anabolic response from strength training is as close to the fountain of youth as we can get. Cardio will not be your main event any longer.

For the next 16 to 20 weeks, flip this thinking to make strength training your first priority. The goal is to strength train at least two days a week. Three days a week is best, two is good, but one time a week won't be enough.

At Results Fitness, we first consider how much time each client has to dedicate to her fitness program. The following guidance will help you design your training schedule according to the time you have available:

• *You have only two or three hours a week.* As your coach, I need you to commit to a minimum of two hours a week. Include the full-body strength training program laid out for you in this book only. These programs offer strength benefits, and you'll get cardiovascular benefits as well by using short rest periods. Your heart will be pumping!

• *You have four hours a week.* Perform three full-body strength workouts along with one high-intensity interval cardio workout. For the cardio-focused workout, I prefer that you use nontraditional cardio tools such as rope intervals, medicine ball slams, or agility ladder work to move in multiple planes of motion, and use a heart rate monitor. I'll lay out the program you can follow in chapter 18.

• *You have five or six hours per week.* Adding in lower-intensity aerobic workouts is optional and necessary only if you are extremely sedentary. Keep an eye on your steps each day to determine whether some extra activity should be a part of your program.

• *You have more than six hours per week to dedicate to your fitness training.* More than six hours of training is a lot, and you'll need to assess your recovery if you'll be going beyond that. Extra activity could be beneficial or could end up being counterproductive. (See the sidebar "NEAT and Adaptations" in chapter 2 for further explanation.)

More Is Not Always Better

Researchers (Hunter et al. 2013) assigned 72 women aged 60 to 74 to one of three groups for 16 weeks:

- Group one did one day of strength training and one day of aerobic training (1+1)
- Group two did two days of strength training and two days of aerobic training (2+2)
- Group three did three days of strength training and three days of aerobic training (3+3)

Interestingly, the 3+3 group didn't get better results than the 2+2 group because the total energy expenditure and activity-related energy expenditure ended up increasing in the 2+2 group but not in the 3+3 group.

The 2+2 group increased their non-exercise caloric burn by 1,400 calories per week, while the 3+3 group actually decreased their non-exercise caloric burn by 1,050 calories per week. That's a difference of 2,450 calories per week, or about a pound of fat every 10 days. While the exact mechanisms as to what caused the differences are unclear, it may be that the 3+3 group was fatigued from doing six workouts a week, so they ended up doing less activity overall.

What do I mean by counterproductive? If you are training too much, you'll end up being less active because your body is tired and needs recovery. I'm sure you've heard the recommendation to get 10,000 steps a day. This number is a good benchmark for an active daily life, but it is not a magic number. Instead, keep track of your steps to see how you improve while making sure you're recovering. Keeping an eye on your steps and how active you are will let you know if your training is becoming too much. Most phones will even track your steps if you don't have a smartwatch. Rule of thumb: If you're going to be doing more than four to six hours of training per week, track your daily activity to ensure it's not decreasing so that adding the extra workouts equals less overall. Don't keep adding training sessions only to end up sitting and napping a whole lot more.

To ensure you're not piling on too much training, anything over six hours will need to be lower intensity to help improve recovery. This can also be known as "living an active lifestyle," like I talked about earlier. For these hours, I recommend doing things you enjoy! Go for a hike, ride your bike, go swimming, enjoy pickleball, play golf, play tennis, or do whatever active hobby you want to spend your time doing. Get out and enjoy an active life!

PRINCIPLE 2: BUILD A FOUNDATION OF MOVING WELL

Gray Cook, founder of the functional movement screen, said "Move well, then move often." The first phase of the strength training program will be the foundation for the rest of the program. This first program is designed to undo some of life's work, addressing common imbalances, weaknesses, and tight muscles so you can move and breath properly with everything engaged.

Over years of sitting too much, wearing improper shoes, and in general not moving enough, certain muscles don't get used often while others get short or tight, and your overall range of motion decreases. Even if you go to the gym regularly, the tendency is to overwork certain areas and movements while neglecting others.

The first step to aging strong is to improve the quality of your movement. The base phase of training has stretches and basic movements, including postural, core, and bodyweight moves to engage all the right muscles. It's always a good idea to go back to basics, so I encourage everyone to complete this phase of the program, even if you're experienced with strength training.

Really take your time going through this first phase. You might feel the exercises are really simple or easy, but I bet you'll find they're anything but. Some of the exercises in this base phase are the hardest you'll do, as we get the right muscles engaged to be able to load heavier weight in later phases.

You will use a warm-up to start each workout throughout every phase. The warm-up not only increases your body temperature as a typical warm-up does but also activates the right muscles, improves range of motion, and improves your quality of movement to fully prepare you for the workout. We call our warm-up RAMP, which stands for this:

Range of motion

Activation

Movement **P**reparation

PRINCIPLE 3: BUILD A BALANCED BODY

The programs in this book will build a balanced body. They take into account the usual imbalances we see when women in their 40s or older start a fitness program and are designed to help prevent injuries and lead you to reach your potential to age strong. I am not a doctor or medical professional of any kind; I am a personal trainer who over the years has seen amazing improvements with certain conditions. If you do have an injury or any of the things discussed in this section, please consult a medical professional before following this program.

Some of the common imbalances these programs will help to correct include the following:

- *Tight hip flexors.* If you've spent a good amount of time sitting over your lifetime, then short hip flexors are most likely going to need to be addressed. This will be one of the first stretches you'll do in your warm-up, along with several exercises to actively stretch the hip flexors while activating the opposite muscle (more on that later). When the hip flexors are short, the hips are hiked forward and the posterior chain (butt and hamstrings) cannot work as well.

- *Quad dominance.* Being more quad dominant than hip dominant means you are stronger on the fronts of your thighs and tend to use these muscles more while neglecting or not being able to fully use the muscles running along the backs of your legs, including your butt and hamstrings. A case of "gluteal amnesia" is not uncommon at this point in life, meaning you are simply unable to use your glute muscles as well as you could. If you look at your body in profile in the mirror and you don't have a round backside, we may need to activate those glute muscles to start doing some work. This isn't just for aesthetics. Being quad dominant can lead to overuse knee injuries such as tendinitis or ACL tears, which happen four to six times more often in women than in men (The Female ACL 2016). As we age, stepping downhill or going down stairs can become one of the things we're least confident doing because "our knees can't handle it." Strengthening the posterior chain by using your glutes when you step up and down will keep your knees tracking properly and strong in these eccentric movements. These programs will help you to build a strong, developed, and shapely butt that is ready to lift weights, climb mountains, ride, run, or do whatever other activities you enjoy in life.

- *Poor posture.* Over time, posture tends to become slumped forward, whether you've spent too much time on the computer, in the car, or just sitting. I know as I approached 40, my lifestyle had become more sedentary because I spent more time seated at my desk than I had in my 20s. A forward head posture will improve with the movements and exercises in this program. You'll find that the stress and tension you carry in your shoulders and neck will decrease, thereby reducing the risk of injury to the neck and upper back.

- *Tight ankles and calves.* Over time, improper footwear causes many people to have tight ankles and calves that don't work as well as they could. These problems can come from wearing high heels or wearing shoes with too much cushion that don't require your feet, ankles, and calves to work as much. The problem is that tight ankles and weak calves can cause issues further up the chain as the body compensates, leading to knee and low-back injuries. Improving range of motion at the ankles, using a foam roller, and doing some balancing exercises along with wearing proper footwear will help reverse some of these problems.

  • *Poor core strength and a lack of low-back stability.* These issues are extremely common in women over 40. They may be caused by too many crunches over the years and not enough stability exercises, along with sitting too much. This is not just about having six-pack abs; in fact, it's really nothing to do with that. All movement originates in the core. The core is not just the abs; it includes the hips, pelvis, abdominals, lower back, mid back, and neck—basically everything but the arms and legs. In this program, you'll see a range of exercises for stabilizing the core (always early in the program) as a priority. Women have wider hips than men do and usually more of an anterior pelvic tilt, meaning the top of their hips is tilted forward, creating tension in their low back and often causing back pain. Strengthening the core will help. Doing these exercises properly will improve everything else. As your core is able to stabilize, you'll be stronger in other movements.

  • *Pelvic floor issues.* After having babies and experiencing hormonal change, many women find their pelvic floor becomes more lax, which can lead to several embarrassing problems, including urinary incontinence or a pelvic floor disorder called prolapse, in which the organs in the pelvis, such as the uterus, fall down and protrude. Both can be avoided by strengthening the pelvic floor muscles, which will improve with strength training. Throughout this program, during the core stability exercises I'll give you cues to engage your deep abdominal and pelvic floor muscles.

PRINCIPLE 4: KEEP THE GOAL THE GOAL

The goal of this program is for you to become strong as you age. It will cycle training volume and intensity to peak at the end of the 16 to 20 weeks. By the final phase, you should be able to complete the baseline tests that follow to be considered aging strong. The plan is laid out for you. All you have to do is stick to the plan and trust the process.

Having a plan that is periodized over time, cycling the exercise demands to keep the body from stalling in your progress to achieve the desired result, is an important concept to understand. If you deviate from the plan or add in your own extra workouts or exercises, the result most likely will not be the same. If you do want to add extra workouts or exercises, my question is, What is your goal? Let's keep the goal the goal and stay focused on doing only the things necessary to get to where we want to go. This plan will do that, I promise. Nothing extra is needed.

Sometimes clients make mistakes by deviating from the plan, often without even realizing it. Common mistakes include the following:

- *Using the same weights, no matter what the rep range is.* You will need a fully equipped gym to properly perform these workouts and stick to the plan. Loading is a key factor to getting the results you desire. If you aren't lifting enough weight, this plan will not get you to the goal.

- *Trying to go hard every workout.* When you start a new phase, I recommend following the plan to do only one or two sets with lighter weights so you can learn the movement. Start with a lower volume week to give your body some extra recovery. You might feel like you could do more on these workout days. Don't. Leave something in the tank on these de-load weeks. If you continually push your body, adding more on top of more, your body will eventually make you take a break. You'll end up injured or sick and set back your training. You can avoid this by following the plan and including a de-load week every four to six weeks.

- *Trying to improve everything at once.* The program in this book is a plan to get you strong. If you decide to also try to improve your endurance while you're following this program, you won't get the same results. Make strength your number one priority for 16 weeks. I promise you'll find that your endurance will improve as you become stronger and more efficient. Once you finish this program, you can set the goal to improve your endurance: Do a triathlon or run your first marathon, I support all that! And we'll get there. For the next 16 weeks, though, focus only on getting strong.

PRINCIPLE 5: CHOOSE HIGH-BENEFIT EXERCISES

You won't see any exercises in this program that isolate any one muscle group. Instead, you'll be doing compound exercises that use a lot of different muscle groups, burn a ton of calories, and get more done at once.

You also won't see any seated stationary strength machine exercises, because every exercise you do as part of this program will give you the most benefit possible by engaging your core to stabilize, working in multiple planes of motion, and overall giving you the highest return for your training in the least amount of time.

Every program is a total-body program. Your exercises will be done in a circuit style with an upper-body exercise paired with a lower-body exercise. This will help you keep your rest periods short while providing time for muscles to rest. While performing your upper-body exercise, your lower body will have a longer rest, and vice versa. Having shorter rests also creates a cardiovascular benefit as you move from one exercise to the next while keeping your intensity high, lifting enough weight to gain strength. It's the best of everything!

Each exercise has a number and a letter. Exercises with the same letter are a pair, and you'll perform them as a circuit for the desired number of reps and sets, performing 1A for 15 reps, then 1B for 15 reps, then repeating 1A again for 2 or 3 sets before moving on to 2A and 2B.

You'll also notice core and power development exercises as a priority. Power is one of the first things we lose as we age, so I put it early in the workouts to make sure you're fresh and able to perform these exercises with high quality.

PRINCIPLE 6: INTENSITY OVER DURATION EQUALS RESULTS

As we age, workouts that focus on intensity rather than long-duration, steady-state exercise will create the hormonal response to build muscle and encourage anti-aging. Each workout needs to be at an intensity that will create a metabolic disturbance. Pushing just outside of what's comfortable will get you the results you want. By working at a high intensity, you'll get what's called excess postexercise oxygen consumption (EPOC); this means that following the workout, your muscles will continue to take up excess oxygen and burn more calories, continuing to provide a benefit before returning to a resting level of metabolic function. You'll burn more calories even while you sleep! Over time, this postexercise effect will lead to dramatic improvements. Usually, after an intense workout that has created this postexercise effect, you'll feel warm the rest of the day because your body temperature remains elevated. With every training session, your goal is to work at an intensity that will create this effect, stoking your metabolism for the next 24 to 48 hours. Who says our metabolism has to slow down as we age? Not if we're ready to push ourselves in the gym!

Because the number of reps will stay the same in each phase, the only way to increase intensity is by lifting more weight or progressing the exercise to a harder version. How much should you lift? Great question! Start light and increase every time. It's also OK to increase within the same workout. At the end of each set, ask yourself, "How many more reps could I have done?" If the answer is five or more, increase the weight for the next set. If the answer is one or two, then stick with that same weight.

At the end of each phase, you'll do a test set on your final set of each exercise. You will perform AMRAP, which stands for "as many reps as possible" to see how many more reps you can actually get. For example, if your program called for 10 reps, but you were able to complete 15 on the final set while using 30-pound dumbbells, you would know you are lifting too light and need to increase your load. Compare your reps to table 13.2 to determine how much weight you should be lifting. In this example, you would scan across the top to the number of reps you got of 15 and look down that column for the amount of weight you lifted (30 pounds [14 kg]). The table shows you could have lifted 35 pounds [16 kg] for 10 reps, which is what you will use from now on.

TABLE 13.2 Repetition Maximum Conversion Chart

Reps	2	3	4	5	6	8	10	12	15
1RM	93%	90%	87%	85%	82%	75%	70%	65%	60%
10	9	9	9	9	8	8	7	7	6
20	19	18	17	17	16	15	14	13	12
30	28	27	26	26	25	23	21	20	18
40	37	36	35	34	33	30	28	26	24
50	47	45	44	43	41	38	35	33	30
60	56	54	52	51	49	45	42	39	36
70	65	63	61	60	57	53	49	46	42
80	74	72	70	68	66	60	56	52	48
90	84	81	78	77	74	68	63	59	54
100	93	90	87	85	82	75	70	65	60
110	102	99	96	94	90	83	77	72	66
120	112	108	104	102	96	90	84	78	72
130	121	117	113	111	107	98	91	85	78
140	130	126	122	119	115	105	98	91	84
150	140	135	131	128	123	113	105	95	90
160	149	144	139	136	131	120	112	104	96
170	158	153	148	145	139	128	119	111	102
180	167	162	157	153	148	135	126	117	108
190	177	171	165	162	156	143	133	124	114
200	186	180	174	170	164	150	140	130	120
210	195	189	183	179	172	158	147	137	126
220	205	198	191	187	180	165	154	143	132
230	214	207	200	196	189	173	161	150	138
240	223	216	209	204	197	180	168	156	144
250	233	225	218	213	205	188	175	163	150
260	242	234	226	221	213	195	182	169	156
270	251	243	235	230	221	203	189	176	162
280	260	252	244	238	230	210	196	182	168
290	270	261	252	247	238	215	203	189	174
300	279	270	261	255	246	225	210	195	180
310	288	279	270	264	254	233	217	202	186
320	298	288	278	272	262	240	224	208	192
330	307	297	287	281	271	245	231	215	196
340	316	306	296	289	279	255	238	221	204
350	326	315	305	295	287	263	245	228	210

(continued)

TABLE 13.2   Repetition Maximum Conversion Chart *(continued)*

Reps	2	3	4	5	6	8	10	12	15
360	335	324	313	306	295	270	252	234	216
370	344	333	322	315	303	278	259	241	222
380	353	342	331	323	312	285	266	247	228
390	363	351	339	332	320	293	273	254	234
400	372	360	348	340	328	300	280	260	240
410	381	369	357	349	336	308	287	267	246
420	391	378	365	357	344	315	294	273	252
430	400	387	374	366	353	323	301	280	258
440	409	396	383	374	361	330	308	285	264
450	419	405	392	383	369	338	315	293	270
460	428	414	400	391	377	345	322	299	276
470	437	423	409	400	385	353	329	306	282
480	446	432	415	408	394	360	336	312	288
490	456	441	426	417	402	368	343	319	294
500	465	450	435	425	410	375	350	325	300
510	474	459	444	434	418	383	357	332	306
520	484	468	452	442	426	390	364	338	312
530	493	477	461	451	435	395	371	345	318
540	502	486	470	459	443	405	378	351	324
550	512	495	479	468	451	413	385	358	330
560	521	504	487	476	459	420	392	364	336

PRINCIPLE 7: CONSISTENCY IS KEY

If there is one factor that will guarantee results, it's showing up every day and being consistent. It's always easy to start a new habit, but it's not always easy to continue the habit as part of your life. To reach your potential as you age, commit to being consistent with your training day after day, week after week, for the rest of your life. This book has a scientific program laid out for you, removing the guesswork, but without consistency, it won't do you any good to help you age strong.

In each phase, you'll alternate two strength workouts, workout A and workout B. If you're training the recommended three times per week, your schedule will look similar to table 13.3. With this schedule, you'll complete each workout six times per month, which is an ideal frequency. At this point, you'll be ready to move to the next phase.

If you are strength training only twice a week, it will take you 6 weeks to get the desired exposures to each workout; instead of a 16-week program, you will take 20 weeks. This is perfectly acceptable and will still get you very good results. Each phase will look like the one in table 13.4.

If you can work out only two days a week, use the program shown in table 13.4. If you find you could add another workout day to your week, add another strength training day, following the pattern shown in table 13.3. If you find you have the time to work out four days a week, you can add a metabolic interval workout as shown in table 13.5.

TABLE 13.3   Three Strength Workouts per Week

Monday	Tuesday	Wednesday	Thursday	Friday	Saturday	Sunday
Workout A		Workout B		Workout A		
Workout B		Workout A		Workout B		
Workout A		Workout B		Workout A		
Workout B		Workout A		Workout B		

TABLE 13.4   Two Strength Workouts per Week

Monday	Tuesday	Wednesday	Thursday	Friday	Saturday	Sunday
Workout A			Workout B			
Workout A			Workout B			
Workout A			Workout B			
Workout A			Workout B			
Workout A			Workout B			
Workout A			Workout B			

TABLE 13.5   Three Strength Workouts and One Metabolic Interval Workout per Week (Maximum Number of Sessions)

Monday	Tuesday	Wednesday	Thursday	Friday	Saturday	Sunday
Workout A		Workout B		Workout A	Metabolic interval	
Workout B		Workout A		Workout B	Metabolic interval	
Workout A		Workout B		Workout A	Metabolic interval	
Workout B		Workout A		Workout B	Metabolic interval	
Workout A		Workout B		Workout A	Metabolic interval	
Workout B		Workout A		Workout B	Metabolic interval	

PRINCIPLE 8: STRONGER EVERY WORKOUT

If your workouts are done right, you'll be stronger, fitter, and ready for more following recovery from the workout, which means the next time you do the workout to create a new demand, you'll need to lift heavier, do more, or tackle a harder variation. This doesn't mean to increase every exercise. Adding weight to an earlier exercise will affect the exercises following it. Make it a goal to bump up the load on one to three exercises each time you work out. The only way to make progress is to progressively increase your weights. If you're not getting stronger, you're not making progress. Many women have a hard time pushing themselves and lifting more weight. Learning to push yourself to do more each workout is a huge part of the success of this program. Learning to grind out one last rep is important to gaining strength as you age. The programs will help you learn that; the plus set at the end of each phase will help you realize how much you are capable of.

On the flip side, be careful not to do more than you're ready for. Throughout the program, I include some skipping, jumping, and other movements that may be too challenging if you have a weak pelvic floor. If you notice that you might be leaking during some of the movements, that is a sign of a weak pelvic floor. Pay extra attention to diaphragmatic breathing and perform the core exercises properly while scaling back the jumping exercises to a lower-impact option until you feel confident that you won't have a problem. This is common, and you don't have to be embarrassed.

How heavy is heavy? You have strength standards to shoot for by the end of the program to give you an idea of what you're working up to. Keep those in mind as you build up. If you're nowhere near them, test yourself on the final plus set of each phase to see if you've been lifting too light.

PRINCIPLE 9: SAME MOVEMENTS AND REP RANGE FOR FOUR TO SIX WEEKS

Your body will adapt to the exercise selection last. You don't need new exercises every workout. Yes, we want to put new demands on our body every workout but sticking with the same reps and exercises for four to six weeks as laid out will give you a chance to master the movements and see yourself progress while increasing the load for the reps in that phase. Focus on progressing your loads each workout while keeping the exercises and reps the same within a phase. This way, when you are ready for a new phase, it will be a brand-new stimulus in a new rep range with different intensity. Again, you may not change every exercise from phase to phase since your body will adapt to the exercise selection last.

In addition, pay attention to the tempo for each exercise, which tells you how fast to do the reps. You'll see the following tempos in the program:

Slow: Lower the weight under control, definite pause, lift the weight under control

Moderate: Lower the weight under control, definite pause, lift the weight as quickly as possible

Fast: Lower the weight quickly, no pause, lift the weight as quickly as possible

X: Lower the weight quickly, no pause, explode the weight up

PRINCIPLE 10: SUPPORT AND ACCOUNTABILITY

You'll do best if you find a good training partner to go through this program with you. Most people are motivated through external accountability. Having somebody else whom you will let down if you don't show up for your workout will make a big difference to your consistency, unless you're one of the rare people who is self-motivated. Having support is key to keeping your motivation to stick to the plan.

I think this is one of our secrets at Results Fitness; everyone works out in small groups. All training sessions are semiprivate, so our clients work out with one or two other people. Having a peer group and a coach, they tend to work harder and feed off each other's energy. Nobody wants to let the group down. "It's easy to quit when you're by yourself, but not when you're with others," one of our clients shared.

PRINCIPLE 11: YOU GET RESULTS FROM YOUR RECOVERY, NOT FROM THE WORKOUT

Give your body time between workouts to recover, regenerate, and rebuild. This is key to getting results. More is not always better. If you're an endurance junkie, be careful not to run off all the hard work you did in the gym lifting weights. Those muscles need time to repair before training again. Extra training can be beneficial but can also be very counterproductive.

Take 24 hours off between training sessions and one day completely off a week. Three days a week of strength training done with an intense effort will be the most you'll be able to handle and recover from if you're doing it right. Sleep is extremely important to your recovery, along with adequate nutrition and hydration. Movement can be as good as active recovery and includes low-intensity exercise and stretching along with modalities such as a foam roller or massage gun to improve tissue quality between sessions. Take your recovery as seriously as you take your training.

Also, if you have a tendency to move through your workout quickly without rest between sets, you're probably not lifting at the intensity you need to be to get the best results. You will need recovery between exercises if your loading is challenging enough.

PRINCIPLE 12: USE A HEART RATE MONITOR FOR METABOLIC INTERVAL SESSIONS

Cardio is a side dish on this program, and when you are going to do it, do not waste your time. Let's do it right. You'll be doing metabolic interval-style cardio sessions. As you are ready to add in the fourth workout session per week of a metabolic interval workout, I highly recommend you use a heart rate monitor to track your intensity and get to know what you're capable of. You'll also be able to track your progress as you get into better shape; your heart rate will recover faster, and it will take you longer to get your work interval to the 85 percent of max heart rate we're shooting for.

A heart rate monitor will customize your cardio session individualized so it is not a generic time-based program. If you don't have a heart rate monitor, you can use the descriptions that follow to check your intensity based on how much you can carry on a conversation.

First, establish the percentages of your max heart rate. These will be used to target the level of effort for every metabolic cardio workout. If you do not currently have or do not plan to purchase and train with a heart rate monitor, use perceived exertion to understand and recognize training intensity. If you are going to train with a monitor, read the information about perceived exertion, then continue to the discussion of using a monitor.

For each workout, use the perceived effort, or "how hard does it feel," chart (figure 13.1) to determine the proper training intensity. You'll be pushing into the red effort, then recovering until you are in the green range.

	Warm-up	Light (recovery range)	Moderate	Hard
% of max heart rate	Under 50%	50-75%	75-85%	85% or more
Rate of perceived exertion (RPE)	Could sing a song.	Go-all-day kind of intensity. Conversations are comfortable.	Can maintain intensity for only a few minutes. Can manage only one or two words in conversation.	Uncomfortable. Able to maintain intensity for only a minute or less. Basic grunts.

FIGURE 13.1 Perceived effort.

If you are going to train with a heart rate monitor, you can establish your heart rate intensity percentages using your age and plugging it into a formula. This is an estimate and will give you an idea of where you should be, but it is based on age, so it could be off if you're in better shape than the average person your age.

Figuring Out Your Heart Rate

You will need to do a bit of math to find the correct beats per minute for each percentage range. This is not difficult, but it does require a couple of days to establish. Use the monitor every morning before you sit up and get out of bed to determine your resting heart rate.

Record the lowest HR reading for five days and then take the average. This is your resting heart rate (RHR).

Once you have your RHR, you're ready to plug it into a simple equation. Subtract your age from 220. From this number, subtract your RHR. Multiply the resulting number (known as your heart rate reserve, or HRR) by the percentages in each range, then add the RHR back in.

For example, let's consider a 45-year-old female with a resting heart rate of 55:

220 – 45 (age) = 175

175 – 55 (RHR) = 120 (HRR)

120 × 0.50 = 60 + 55 (RHR) = 115 beats per minute at the top of the warm-up range

120 × 0.75 = 90 + 55 (RHR) = 145 beats per minute at the top of the recovery range

120 × 0.85 = 102 + 55 (RHR) = 157 beats per minute at the bottom of the work interval (hard max effort) range

Write your results into figure 13.2 to create your own personal intensity zone.

	Warm-up	Light (recovery range)	Moderate	Hard
% of max heart rate	Under 50%	50-75%	75-85%	85% or more
Rate of perceived exertion (RPE)	Could sing a song.	Go-all-day kind of intensity. Conversations are comfortable.	Can maintain intensity for only a few minutes. Can manage only one or two words in conversation.	Uncomfortable. Able to maintain intensity for only a minute or less. Basic grunts.
My beats per minute				

FIGURE 13.2 Personal intensity zone.

CONCLUSION

This chapter should help you understand the principles that the programs in this book are built on. These are not random, thrown-together programs. They are based on solid scientific principles and give you the most effective best programming for a woman in her 40s and beyond. Now, let's get to work!

CHAPTER 14

THE BASE PHASE

This first phase is home base. In this phase, you'll set yourself up for success for the rest of the program. Take your time going through these exercises, really engaging the right muscles, and reading the descriptions from the earlier chapters to get the cues right.

In this initial phase, start with light weights and then progress from there. At the end of each set, ask yourself, "How many more reps could I have done?" If the answer is five or more, increase the weight for the next set. If the answer is one or two, then stick with that same weight.

In addition, pay attention to the tempo for each exercise, which tells you how fast to do the reps. You'll see the following tempos in the program:

Slow: Lower the weight under control, definite pause, lift the weight under control

Moderate: Lower the weight under control, definite pause, lift the weight as quickly as possible

X: Lower the weight quickly, no pause, explode the weight up

BASE PHASE RAMP

Foam roll the quadriceps, adductors, mid to upper back, and hips (page 86): 30 to 60 seconds on each area

Positional breathing reset (page 93): 6 deep breaths

Two-leg hip bridge (page 97): 10 reps

Half-kneeling hip flexor mobility (page 94): Hold for 30 to 60 seconds each leg

Windshield wiper 90/90 hip stretch (page 95): 5 each direction

In-place Spiderman on incline (page 100): 5 each side

Side-lying rib pull (page 104): 5 each side

Open half-kneeling ankle mobility (page 108): 4 each ankle

Bodyweight prisoner RDL (page 115): 4 reps

Tall kneel to half kneel (page 118): 4 each leg

Lateral squat (page 122): 4 each direction

Suspension trainer squat prying (page 125): 5 each side

High-knee march in place (page 129): 20 sec

Linear skip (page 131): 20 sec

BASE PHASE: WORKOUT A

1A Front Plank (page 138)

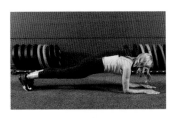

Sets: 2
Reps, weeks 1-4: 1
Tempo: 30-45 sec hold
Rest: 30 sec

1B Cable Half-Kneeling Anti-Rotation Press (page 146)

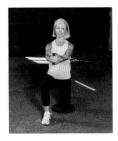

Sets: 2
Reps, weeks 1-3: 12-15 each side
Reps, week 4: 12-15 each side for the first set, then AMRAP on the second set
Tempo: Slow
Rest: 60 sec

2A Medicine Ball Floor Slam (page 186)

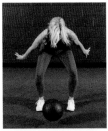

Sets: 2
Reps, weeks 1-4: 6
Tempo: X
Rest: 60 sec

3A Kettlebell Goblet Squat (page 168)

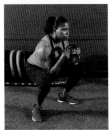

Sets: 2
Reps, weeks 1-3: 12-15
Reps, week 4: 12-15 for the first set, then AMRAP on the second set
Tempo: Moderate
Rest: 30 sec

3B Cable Half-Kneeling One-Arm Row (page 156)

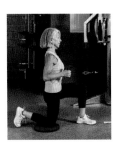

Sets: 2
Reps, weeks 1-3: 12-15
Reps, week 4: 12-15 for the first set, then AMRAP on the second set
Tempo: Moderate
Rest: 60 sec

(continued)

BASE PHASE: WORKOUT A *(continued)*

4A Sandbag Staggered-Stance RDL (page 173)

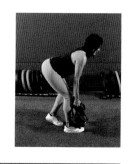

Sets: 2

Reps, weeks 1-3: 12-15

Reps, week 4: 12-15 for the first set, then AMRAP on
the second set

Tempo: Moderate

Rest: 60 sec

4B Incline Push-Up (page 154)

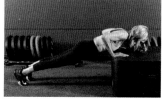

Sets: 2

Reps, weeks 1-3: 12-15

Reps, week 4: 12-15 for the first set, then
AMRAP on the second set

Tempo: Moderate

Rest: 60 sec

5A Battle Rope Intervals (page 204)

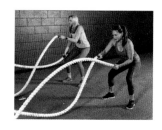

Sets: 3

Reps: 30 sec

Tempo: X

Rest: 60 sec

BASE PHASE: WORKOUT B

1A Hollow Hold (page 144)

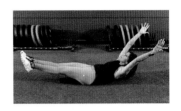

Sets: 2

Reps, weeks 1-4: 1

Tempo: 20-30 sec hold

Rest: 30 sec

1B Cable Tall-Kneeling Anti-Rotation Press (page 146)

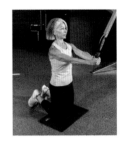

Sets: 2

Reps, weeks 1-3: 12-15 each side

Reps, week 4: 12-15 each side for the first set, then AMRAP on the second set

Tempo: Slow

Rest: 60 sec

2A Medicine Ball Tall-Kneeling Chest Throw (page 182)

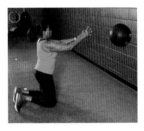

Sets: 2

Reps, weeks 1-4: 6

Tempo: X

Rest: 60 sec

3A Kettlebell Deadlift (page 177)

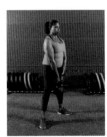

Sets: 2

Reps, weeks 1-3: 12-15

Reps, week 4: 12-15 for the first set, then AMRAP on the second set

Tempo: Moderate

Rest: 30 sec

3B Dumbbell Incline Bench Press (page 165)

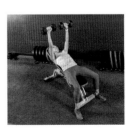

Sets: 2

Reps, weeks 1-3: 12-15

Reps, weeks 4: 12-15 for the first set, then AMRAP on the second set

Tempo: Moderate

Rest: 60 sec

(continued)

BASE PHASE: WORKOUT B *(continued)*

4A Step-Up (page 172)

Sets: 2

Reps, weeks 1-3: 12-15

Reps, week 4: 12-15 for the first set, then AMRAP on
the second set

Tempo: Moderate

Rest: 30 sec

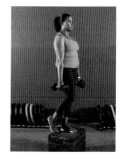

4B Cable Tall-Kneeling Neutral-Grip Pull-Down (page 158)

Sets: 2

Reps, weeks 1-3: 12-15

Reps, week 4: 12-15 for the first set, then AMRAP on
the second set

Tempo: Moderate

Rest: 60 sec

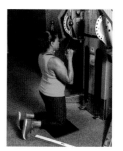

5A Fan Bike Sprint (page 207)

Sets: 3

Reps: 30 sec

Tempo: X

Rest: 60 sec

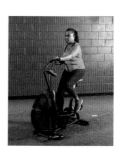

CONCLUSION

Congratulations on completing the base phase! After following this phase
for four to six weeks, you'll notice yourself moving better, improving your
mobility and strength. In the next phase, you'll be performing lower reps
with heavier weights using this new strength and mobility. The exercises
will progress, and you'll have all new demands on your body.

CHAPTER 15

THE BUILD PHASE

Now that you've completed the base phase, you're ready to drop the number of reps as you increase the load and build some serious strength and muscle. Remember: We're not afraid of gaining muscle. We're afraid of losing muscle! Let's lift some heavy weights during this phase. Refer to the exercise descriptions in the previous chapters to make sure you are performing the workout with good form and are following all the cues.

In this phase, bump your weights up as your reps are going down. At the end of each set, ask yourself, "How many more reps could I have done?" If the answer is five or more, increase the weight for the next set. If the answer is one or two, then stick with that weight.

In addition, pay attention to the tempo for each exercise, which tells you how fast to do the reps. You'll see the following tempos in the program:

Slow: Lower the weight under control, definite pause, lift the weight under control

Moderate: Lower the weight under control, definite pause, lift the weight as quickly as possible

X: Lower the weight quickly, no pause, explode the weight up

BUILD PHASE RAMP

Foam roll the quadriceps, adductors, mid to upper back, and hips (page 86): 30 to 60 seconds on each area

Positional breathing reset (page 93): 6 deep breaths

Bridge with march (page 102): 10 reps

Hip flexor mobility with one-arm reach (page 96): 6 each side

Frog stretch (page 98): 5 reps

In-place Spiderman on floor (page 100): 5 each side

Heel sit quadruped thoracic spine external rotation (page 105): 5 reps each side

Floor pike alternating ankle mobility (page 109): 4 each ankle

Bodyweight staggered-stance RDL (page 116): 4 each leg

Suspension trainer stationary split squat (page 120): 4 each leg

Alternating lateral squat (page 123): 4 each side

Toe touch to frog squat (page 126): 5 reps

Drop to base (page 133): 5 reps

Sprint in place (page 135): 10 sec

BUILD PHASE: WORKOUT A

1A Alternating One-Leg Front Plank (page 139)

Sets: 2
Reps, weeks 1-4: 6 each leg
Tempo: 5 sec hold
Rest: 30 sec

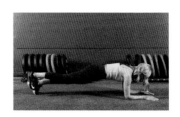

1B Glute Bridge With Cable Core Activation (page 140)

Sets: 2
Reps, weeks 1-4: 6-8
Tempo: Moderate
Rest: 60 sec

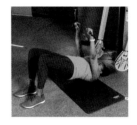

2A Medicine Ball Half-Kneeling Chop Throw (page 184)

Sets 2
Reps, weeks 1-4: 6-8
Tempo: X
Rest: 60 sec

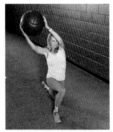

3A Kettlebell Goblet Squat (page 168)

Sets: 2
Reps, weeks 1-3: 6-8
Reps, week 4: 6-8 for the first set, then AMRAP on
  the second set
Tempo: Moderate
Rest: 30 sec

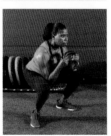

3B Suspension Trainer Inverted Neutral-Grip Row (page 163)

Sets: 2
Reps, weeks 1-3: 6-8
Reps, week 4: 6-8 for the first set, then AMRAP on
  the second set
Tempo: Moderate
Rest: 60 sec

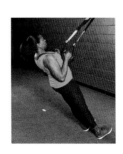

(continued)

BUILD PHASE: WORKOUT A *(continued)*

4A Kettlebell Staggered-Stance RDL (page 174)

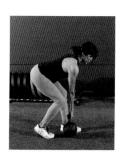

Sets: 2

Reps, weeks 1-3: 6-8

Reps, week 4: 6-8 for the first set, then AMRAP on
the second set

Tempo: Moderate

Rest: 30 sec

4B Dumbbell Half-Kneeling One-Arm Overhead Press (page 164)

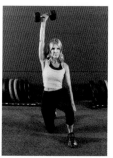

Sets: 2

Reps, weeks 1-3: 6-8

Reps, week 4: 6-8 for the first set, then AMRAP on
the second set

Tempo: Moderate

Rest: 60 sec

5A Fan Bike Sprint (page 207)

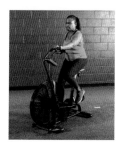

Sets: 4

Reps: 45 sec

Tempo: X

Rest: 60 sec

BUILD PHASE: WORKOUT B

1A Sandbag Dead Bug Alternating-Leg Reach (page 150)

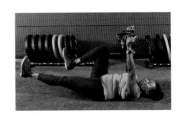

Sets: 2
Reps, weeks 1-4: 6 each side
Tempo: Moderate
Rest: 30 sec

1B Cable Half-Kneeling Lift (page 148)

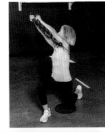

Sets: 2
Reps, weeks 1-4: 6-8
Tempo: Slow
Rest: 60 sec

2A Cable Half-Kneeling One-Arm Row (page 156)

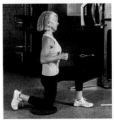

Sets: 2
Reps, weeks 1-4: 6-8 each leg
Tempo: X
Rest: 60 sec

3A Kettlebell Deadlift (page 177)

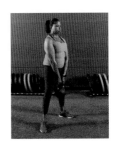

Sets: 2
Reps, weeks 1-3: 6-8
Reps, week 4: 6-8 for the first set, then AMRAP on
    the second set
Tempo: Moderate
Rest: 30 sec

3B Incline Push-Up (page 154)

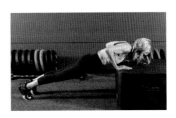

Sets: 2
Reps, weeks 1-3: 6-8
Reps, week 4: 6-8 for the first set, then
    AMRAP on the second set
Tempo: Moderate
Rest: 60 sec

(continued)

BUILD PHASE: WORKOUT B *(continued)*

4A Goblet Split Squat (page 169)

Sets: 2

Reps, weeks 1-3: 6-8

Reps, week 4: 6-8 for the first set, then AMRAP on
the second set

Tempo: Moderate

Rest: 30 sec

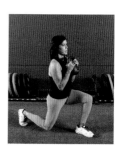

4B Cable Tall-Kneeling Neutral-Grip Pull-Down (page 158)

Sets: 2

Reps, weeks 1-3: 6-8

Reps, week 4: 6-8 for the first set, then AMRAP on
the second set

Tempo: Moderate

Rest: 60 sec

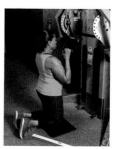

5A Battle Rope Intervals (page 204)

Sets: 4

Reps: 45 sec

Tempo: X

Rest: 90 sec

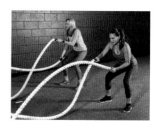

CONCLUSION

Congratulations on completing the build phase, where you have started to learn how to push yourself with some heavier weights and are lifting more than maybe you have before. *That* is how you age strong. In the next phase, the reps will increase as you keep your weights as heavy as you can so you'll progress with the exercises you're doing. You are on the path to getting stronger, fitter, and confident as you age.

CHAPTER 16

THE STRONGER PHASE

Continuing to improve your movement, you're now ready to increase the volume by both increasing the number of reps you perform and the load, along with progressing some of the exercises as you're getting stronger. You'll start to hit some of your benchmarks to age strong. Watch for the goal numbers on the exercises and see what you can do to hit them. Remember to refer to the exercise descriptions in previous chapters to make sure you're performing the workouts with proper form. As you're lifting heavier, it becomes crucial to keep all the coaching cues in mind.

By this phase, your weights should be progressing. Working with a coach or training partner is a great idea to help spot you, push you, and keep an eye on your form as you are getting stronger. At the end of each set, ask yourself, "How many more reps could I have done?" If the answer is five or more, increase the weight for the next set. If the answer is one or two, then stick with that weight.

In addition, pay attention to the tempo for each exercise, which tells you how fast to do the reps. You'll see the following tempos in the program:

Slow: Lower the weight under control, definite pause, lift the weight under control

Moderate: Lower the weight under control, definite pause, lift the weight as quickly as possible

X: Lower the weight quickly, no pause, explode the weight up

STRONGER PHASE RAMP

Foam roll the quadriceps, adductors, mid to upper back, and hips (page 86): 30 to 60 seconds on each area

Positional breathing reset (page 93): 6 deep breaths

One-leg knee hug hip bridge (page 103): 10 each leg

Open half-kneeling position with T-reach (page 107): 6 each side

90/90 stretch (page 99): 5 each direction

Heel sit quadruped alternating reach-through (page 106): 6 each side

Open half-kneeling ankle mobility (page 108): 4 each ankle

World's greatest stretch: lunge with hamstring stretch and T-reach (page 111): 5 each side

Bodyweight one-leg tempo RDL (page 118): 4 each leg

Reverse lunge with rotation (page 121): 4 each leg

Alternating lateral lunge (page 199): 4 each leg

Toe touch to bodyweight squat (page 127): 5 reps

Lateral shuffle (page 130): 4 each direction

Sprint in place (page 135): 10 sec

STRONGER PHASE: WORKOUT A

1A Alternating Arm Reach Front Plank (page 141)

Sets: 2
Reps, weeks 1-4: 6 each side
Tempo: 5 sec hold
Rest: 30 sec

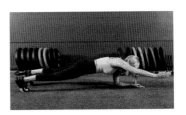

1B Sandbag Full Dead Bug (page 151)

Sets: 2
Reps, weeks 1-4: 10-12 each side
Tempo: Moderate
Rest: 60 sec

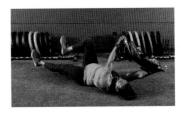

2A Sandbag Clean (page 187)

Sets: 2
Reps, weeks 1-4: 6
Tempo: X
Rest: 60 sec

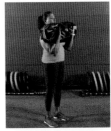

3A Goblet Split Squat (page 169)

Sets: 2
Reps, weeks 1-3: 10-12
Reps, week 4: 10-12 for the first set, then AMRAP on
  the second set
Tempo: Moderate
Rest: 30 sec

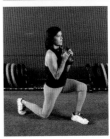

3B Cable Tall-Kneeling Overhand-Grip Pull-Down (page 159)

Sets: 2
Reps, weeks 1-3: 10-12
Reps, week 4: 10-12 for the first set, then AMRAP on
  the second set
Tempo: Moderate
Rest: 60 sec

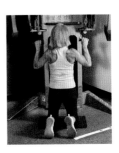

(continued)

STRONGER PHASE: WORKOUT A *(continued)*

4A Sandbag Slider One-Leg RDL (page 175)

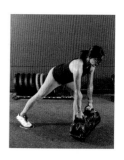

Sets: 2

Reps, weeks 1-3: 10-12

Reps, week 4: 10-12 for the first set, then AMRAP on
the second set

Tempo: Moderate

Rest: 30 sec

4B Dumbbell Half-Kneeling One-Arm Overhead Press (page 164)

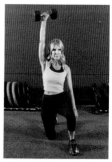

Sets: 2

Reps, weeks 1-3: 10-12

Reps, week 4: 10-12 for the first set, then AMRAP on
the second set

Tempo: Moderate

Rest: 60 sec

5A Fan Bike Sprint (page 207)

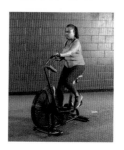

Sets: 4

Reps: 30 sec

Tempo: X

Rest: 60 sec

STRONGER PHASE: WORKOUT B

1A Sandbag Iso Kneeling Side Plank (page 142)

Sets: 2
Reps: 30 sec each side
Tempo: Hold
Rest: 30 sec

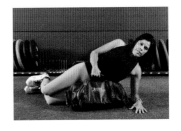

1B Cable Half-Kneeling Lift (page 148)

Sets: 2
Reps, weeks 1-4: 10-12 each side
Tempo: Moderate
Rest: 60 sec

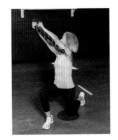

2A Ladder Drill: Forward Two In/Two Out (page 200)

Sets: 2
Reps, weeks 1-4: 20 sec
Tempo: X
Rest: 60 sec

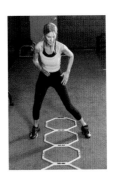

3A High Hex Bar Deadlift (page 178)

Sets: 2
Reps, weeks 1-3: 10-12
Reps, week 4: 10-12 for the first set, then AMRAP on
 the second set
Tempo: Moderate
Rest: 30 sec

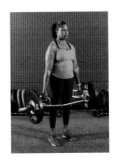

(continued)

STRONGER PHASE: WORKOUT B *(continued)*

3B Incline Push-Up (page 154)

Sets: 2

Reps, weeks 1-3: 10-12

Reps, weeks 4: 10-12 for the first set, then
AMRAP on the second set

Tempo: Moderate

Rest: 60 sec

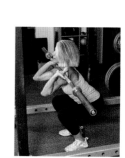

4A Front Squat (page 171)

Sets: 2

Reps, weeks 1-3: 10-12

Reps, week 4: 10-12 for the first set, then AMRAP on
the second set

Tempo: Moderate

Rest: 30 sec

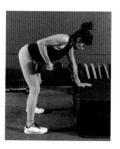

4B Dumbbell Three-Point Neutral-Grip Row (page 161)

Sets: 2

Reps, weeks 1-3: 10-12

Reps, week 4: 10-12 for the first set, then AMRAP on
the second set

Tempo: Moderate

Rest: 60 sec

5A Battle Rope Intervals (page 204)

Sets: 4

Reps: 30 sec

Tempo: X

Rest: 90 sec

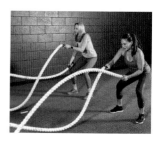

CONCLUSION

Congratulations on completing the stronger phase! You are absolutely getting stronger as you age! In fact, you are reversing the aging process at this point because you are gaining muscle and improving your mobility and strength. You are able to do things you couldn't do when you started. Go you! As you head into the final phase of this program, set some goals to hit some of the baseline standards and surprise yourself with what you can do.

CHAPTER 17

THE AGE STRONG PHASE

In the final phase, you'll hit some baseline strength standards. You'll be able to do exercises such as a push-up and lift a certain amount of weight to finish this program stronger than when you started. Refer to the exercise descriptions in previous chapters to check your form. Learn the proper coaching cues and get the most out of every exercise in this final phase.

Push yourself to hit some personal records (PRs). Working with a coach or training partner is a great idea to help spot you, push you, and keep an eye on your form as you are getting stronger. Simply having someone watching you will make you eke out a heavier weight or one more rep. A qualified coach who gives you feedback will help you get even more out of it. At the end of each set, ask yourself, "How many more reps could I have done?" If the answer is five or more, increase the weight for the next set. If the answer is one or two, then stick with that same weight.

In addition, pay attention to the tempo for each exercise, which tells you how fast to do the reps. You'll see the following tempos in the program:

Slow: Lower the weight under control, definite pause, lift the weight under control

Modcrate: Lower the weight under control, definite pause, lift the weight as quickly as possible

X: Lower the weight quickly, no pause, explode the weight up

AGE STRONG PHASE RAMP

Foam roll the quadriceps, adductors, mid to upper back, and hips (page 86): 30 to 60 seconds on each area

Positional breathing reset (page 93): 6 deep breaths

One-leg knee hug hip bridge (page 103): 10 each leg

Open half-kneeling position with T-reach (page 107): 6 each side

Open half-kneeling windmill (page 112): 5 each direction

Wall ankle mobility drill (page 110): 4 each ankle

Turkish get-up (page 113): 3 each side

Bodyweight one-leg RDL (page 117): 4 each side

Reverse lunge with rotation (page 121): 4 each leg

Low lateral squat (page 123): 4 each side

Toe touch to squat with overhead reach (page 128): 5 reps

Lateral skip (page 132): 4 each direction

Sprint in place (page 135): 10 sec

AGE STRONG PHASE: WORKOUT A

1A Hanging Hollow Hold (goal = 60 sec; page 145)

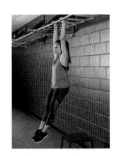

Sets: 2
Reps, weeks 1-4: 1
Tempo: 60 sec hold
Rest: 30 sec

1B Suspension Trainer Prone Jackknife (page 152)

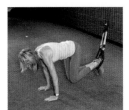

Sets: 2
Reps, weeks 1-4: 5-7
Tempo: Moderate
Rest: 60 sec

2A Cable Horizontal Wood Chop (page 149)

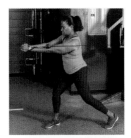

Sets: 2
Reps, weeks 1-4: 5-7 each side
Tempo: X
Rest: 60 sec

3A High Hex Bar Deadlift (goal = 75% of body weight; page 178)

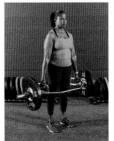

Sets: 2
Reps, weeks 1-3: 5-7
Reps, week 4: 5-7 for the first set, then AMRAP on the second set
Tempo: Moderate
Rest: 30 sec

3B Dumbbell One-Arm Bench Press (page 166)

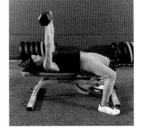

Sets: 2
Reps, weeks 1-3: 5-7
Reps, week 4: 5-7 for the first set, then AMRAP on the second set
Tempo: Moderate
Rest: 60 sec

(continued)

AGE STRONG PHASE: WORKOUT A *(continued)*

4A Goblet Split Squat (goal = 25% of body weight; page 169)

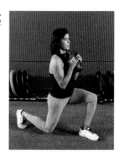

Sets: 2

Reps, weeks 1-3: 5-7

Reps, week 4: 5-7 for the first set, then AMRAP on the
  second set

Tempo: Moderate

Rest: 30 sec

4B Cable Tall-Kneeling Neutral-Grip Pull-Down (page 158)

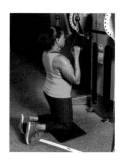

Sets: 2

Reps, weeks 1-3: 5-7

Reps, week 4: 5-7 for the first set, then AMRAP on the
  second set

Tempo: Moderate

Rest: 60 sec

5A Fan Bike Sprint (page 207)

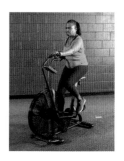

Sets: 4

Reps: 45 sec

Tempo: X

Rest: 60 sec

AGE STRONG PHASE: WORKOUT B

1A Front Plank (goal = 60 sec; page 138)

Sets: 2
Reps, weeks 1-4: 1
Tempo: Hold
Rest: 30 sec

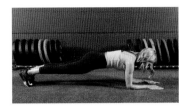

1B Side Plank (goal = 60 sec; page 143)

Sets: 2
Reps, weeks 1-4: 1 each side
Tempo: Hold
Rest: 60 sec

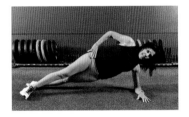

2A Ladder Drill: Forward Two In/Two Out (page 200)

Sets: 3
Reps, weeks 1-4: 60 sec
Tempo: X
Rest: 60 sec

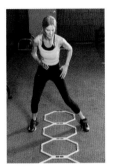

3A Front Squat (goal = 50% of body weight; page 171)

Sets: 2
Reps, weeks 1-3: 5-7
Reps, week 4: 5-7 for the first set, then AMRAP on the second set
Tempo: Moderate
Rest: 30 sec

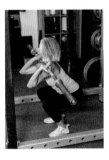

(continued)

AGE STRONG PHASE: WORKOUT B *(continued)*

3B Dumbbell Two-Point Row (goal = 25% of body weight; page 162)

Sets: 2

Reps, weeks 1-3: 5-7

Reps, weeks 4: 5-7 for the first set, then AMRAP on the second set

Tempo: Moderate

Rest: 60 sec

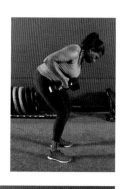

4A Dumbbell One-Leg RDL (goal = 40% of body weight; page 176)

Sets: 2

Reps, weeks 1-3: 5-7

Reps, week 4: 5-7 for the first set, then AMRAP on the second set

Tempo: Moderate

Rest: 30 sec

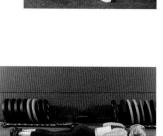

4B Push-Up (add load if you can do more than 6; page 155)

Sets: 2

Reps, weeks 1-3: 5-7

Reps, week 4: 5-7 for the first set, then AMRAP on the second set

Tempo: Moderate

Rest: 60 sec

5A Battle Rope Intervals (page 204)

Sets: 4

Reps: 45 sec

Tempo: X

Rest: 90 sec

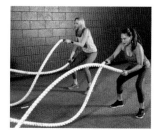

CONCLUSION

Congratulations on completing the final phase of the age strong program. This is only the beginning of your strength training journey. Hopefully you're hooked on feeling strong and are ready to continue your new habit of lifting weights, challenging yourself in the gym and getting stronger as you age.

CHAPTER 18

METABOLIC INTERVAL WORKOUTS

Metabolic interval workouts are a side dish to your strength training programs. If you have four hours or more a week that you can dedicate to training, you'll perform up to two of these workouts a week with your strength sessions, as long as you are recovering properly, getting stronger every strength session, and are able to handle the extra volume. Quality, not quantity of workouts, is most important. Fewer high-quality workouts that you can fully recover from is the goal.

Metabolic interval workouts will boost your metabolism, help improve your cardiovascular fitness, and burn extra calories to achieve the body composition you want. Your first priority is to build base strength, movement, and mobility. Give yourself a couple weeks on the base phase strength program before adding metabolic intervals.

The metabolic workouts will be done interval-style. Your heart rate will increase during the work period—aim for 85 percent of your max heart rate and hold it as long as you can—you will rest until your heart rate returns to below 75 percent of max heart rate and then you'll go again. To elevate your heart rate, move as fast as you can, using as much weight as you can while keeping good form. If you go too light or move at a slow pace, it will take you much longer to elevate your heart rate and lead to a longer, less effective workout.

You'll perform five exercises in a row, each time hitting 85% heart rate with full recovery between each exercise to 75% or less, then complete a full recovery for two to three minutes as needed before repeating the five exercises again.

Phase one, base phase: perform 2 rounds

Phase two, build phase: perform 3 rounds

Phase three, stronger phase: perform 4 rounds

Phase four, age strong phase: perform 5 rounds

THE METABOLIC EXERCISE MENU

Choose one exercise from each of the five groups for each workout.

Group 1: Locomotion

Ladder drills: Hopscotch, Ickey shuffle, two steps/one step, lateral shuffle (page 200)

Jump rope (page 203)

Treadmill sprint or floor sprint (page 208)

Walking lunge (page 195)

Fan bike sprint (page 207)

Stair climber (page 208)

Battle rope intervals (page 204)

Group 2: Core

Mountain climber (page 209)

Medicine ball chest throw (page 183)

Push-up (page 155)

Spiderman (page 211)

Forward crawl with sandbag drag (page 212)

Group 3: Squat

Bodyweight squat (page 191)

Jump squat (page 193)

Burpee or squat thrust (page 194)

Box jump (page 180)

Medicine ball squat thrust (page 194)

Sandbag bear hug squat (page 192)

Group 4: Hinge

Kettlebell swing (page 190)

Alternating kettlebell clean (page 189)

Medicine ball floor slam (page 186)

Medicine ball side throw (page 185)

Sandbag clean and press (page 188)

Group 5: Unilateral

Lunge with rotation (page 196)

Lunge jump (page 197)

Explosive step-up (page 181)

Alternating lateral lunge (page 199)

Sandbag dynamic reverse lunge (page 198)

Sandbag dynamic reverse lunge with rotation (page 198)

CONCLUSION

Congratulations on completing the entire age strong program! This is only the beginning of your journey because you have learned how to improve your strength, health, and fitness. You have the confidence to enjoy more as you age. By this point, you'll be feeling strong and able to do things you never thought you could. In the epilogue, I'll share some final thoughts on aging strong. After that, look around to offer someone you have inspired the chance to join you by recommending this book. I hope you'll keep your copy to use as a reference for a dose of inspiration or a reminder when you need it.

EPILOGUE:
FOCUS AND COMMIT

Don't be afraid of aging. Embrace it. Make the most of it. Follow the recommendations in this book and become stronger, fitter, and healthier as you age. Having a goal gives you a direction and helps you know if you are on the right path or not. Setting and reaching a goal is one thing, but maintaining the goal is everything.

This program is not something you stop doing. You will learn a lot, build new habits, and potentially feel like a different person. Focus on what you can do! Let go of any weight loss goals and steer clear of focusing on changing how you look. Instead, what do you want to be able to do that you couldn't before? What new skills do you want to learn now that you are feeling strong, fit, and athletic?

As you complete the programs in this book and enjoy your newfound strength, you'll keep working on building it! The information in this book is designed with your lifestyle in mind. Become as committed to your new lifestyle as you were to your previous one. With slow changes in daily routines, increases in your strength and confidence, and the reward of a healthy and progressively stronger and fitter body, commitment to your new life will happen. By focusing on building new habits over time, you'll find your goals are easier to maintain.

It's never too late to become the person you always wanted to be. You are the only one to decide what limits are placed on you as you age. For support and inspiration, you can visit my website at rachelcosgrove.com to learn more about connecting with the community of women who are ready to age strong!

REFERENCES

CHAPTER 1

Baena-Garcia, L., M. Flor-Alemany, N. Marín-Jiménez, P. Aranda, and V.A. Aparicio. 2022. "A 16-Week Multicomponent Exercise Training Program Improves Menopause-Related Symptoms in Middle-Aged Women: The FLAMENCO Project Randomized Control Trial." *Menopause* 29 (5): 537-544.

Borde, R., T. Hortobagyi, and U. Granacher. 2015. "Dose-Response Relationships of Resistance Training in Healthy Old Adults: A Systematic Review and Meta-Analysis." *Sports Medicine* 45 (12): 1693-1720.

Centers for Disease Control and Prevention, National Center for Chronic Disease Prevention and Health Promotion, Division of Population Health. 2021. "Arthritis-Related Statistics." www.cdc.gov/arthritis/data_statistics/arthritis-related-stats.htm#print

Chavez, A., R. Scales, and J.M. Kling. 2021. "Promoting Physical Activity in Older Women to Maximize Health." *Cleveland Clinic Journal of Medicine* 88 (7): 405-415.

Cleary, M.P., and M.E. Grossmann. 2009. "Minireview: Obesity and Breast Cancer: The Estrogen Connection." *Endocrinology* 150 (6): 2537-2542.

Crowley, C., and H.S. Lodge, M.D. 2004. *Younger Next Year: Live Strong, Fit and Sexy—Until You're 80 and Beyond*. New York: Workman Publishing.

Cunha, P.M., C.M. Tomeleri, M.A. Nascimento, J.L. Mayhew, E. Fungari, L.T. Cyrino, D.S. Barbosa, D. Venturini, and E.S. Cyrino. 2021. "Comparison of Low and High Volume of Resistance Training on Body Fat and Blood Biomarkers in Untrained Older Women: A Randomized Clinical Trial." *Journal of Strength and Conditioning Research* 35 (1): 1-8. https://pubmed.ncbi.nlm.nih.gov/31306389.

The Female ACL: Why Is It More Prone to Injury? 2016. *Journal of Orthopaedics* 13 (2): A1-A4. https://doi.org/10.1016/S0972-978X(16)00023-4.

Ferrucci, L. 2008. "The Baltimore Longitudinal Study of Aging (BLSA): A 50-Year-Long Journey and Plans for the Future." *The Journals of Gerontology: Series A* 63 (12): 1416-1419. https://doi.org/10.1093/gerona/63.12.1416.

Fragala, M.S., E.L. Cadore, S. Dorgo, M. Izquierdo, W.J. Kraemer, M.D. Peterson, and E.D. Ryan. 2019. "Resistance Training for Older Adults: Position Statement from the National Strength and Conditioning Association." *Journal of Strength and Conditioning Research* 33 (8): 2019-2052.

Gould, L.M., A.N. Gordon, H.E. Cabre, A.T. Hoyle, E.D. Ryan, A.C. Hackney, and A.E. Smith-Ryan. 2022. "Metabolic Effects of Menopause: A Cross-Sectional Characterization of Body Composition and Exercise Metabolism." *Menopause* 29 (4): 377-389. https://doi.org/10.1097/GME.0000000000001932.

Groh, M.M., and J. Herrera. 2009. "A Comprehensive Review of Hip Labrum Tears." *Current Reviews in Musculoskeletal Medicine* 2 (2): 105-117.

Hoff, J., A. Gran, and J. Helgerud. 2002. "Maximal Strength Training Improves Aerobic Endurance Performance." *Scandinavian Journal of Medical Science and Sports* 12 (5): 288-295. https://doi.org/10.1034/j.1600-0838.2002.01140.x.

Hoke, M., N.B. Omar, J.W. Amburgy, D.M. Self, A. Schnell, S.A. Morgan, E. Larios, and M.R. Chambers. 2020. "Impact of Exercise on Bone Mineral Density, Fall Prevention, and Vertebral Fragility Fractures in Postmenopausal Osteoporotic Women." *Journal of Clinical Neuroscience* 76: 261-263.

Hong, A.R., and S.W. Kim. 2018. "Effects of Resistance Exercise on Bone Health." *Endocrinology and Metabolism* 33 (4): 435-444.

Hurkmans, E., F.J. Van Der Giesen, T.P. Vliet Vlieland, J. Schoones, and E.C.H.M. Van den Ende. 2009. "Dynamic Exercise Programs (Aerobic Capacity and/or Muscle Strength Training) in Patients With Rheumatoid Arthritis." *The Cochrane Database of Systematic Reviews* 2009 (4): CD006853.

Kamada, M., E.J. Shiroma, J.E. Buring, M. Miyachi, and I.M. Lee. 2017. Strength Training and All-Cause, Cardiovascular Disease, and Cancer Mortality in Older Women: A Cohort Study. *Journal of the American Heart Association* 6 (11): e007677.

Monash University, Women's Health Research Program. 2023. "Insulin Resistance in the Menopause." www.monash.edu/medicine/sphpm/units/womenshealth/info-4-health-practitioners/insulin-resistance-in-the-menopause.

National Institute on Aging. 2021. "Loneliness and Social Isolation—Tips for Staying Connected." www.nia.nih.gov/health/loneliness-and-social-isolation-tips-staying-connected.

Omoigui, S. 2007. "The Interleukin-6 Inflammation Pathway from Cholesterol to Aging—Role of Statins, Bisphosphonates and Plant Polyphenols in Aging and Age-Related Diseases." *Immunity & Ageing* 4 (1). https://doi.org/10.1186/1742-4933-4-1.

Seguin, R.A., G. Eldridge, W. Lynch, and L.C. Paul. 2013. "Strength Training Improves Body Image and Physical Activity Behaviors Among Midlife and Older Rural Women." *Journal of Extension* 51 (4): 4FEA2.

Sheth, U., D. Wasserstein, R. Jenkinson, and R. Moineddin. 2017. "The Epidemiology and Trends in Management of Acute Achilles Tendon Ruptures in Ontario, Canada." *The Bone & Joint Journal*, January 2017. https://online.boneandjoint.org.uk/doi/full/10.1302/0301-620X.99B1.BJJ-2016-0434.R1.

Taylor, J.L., N.G. Regier, Q. Li, M. Liu, S.L. Szanton, and R.L. Skolasky. 2022. "The Impact of Low Back Pain and Vigorous Activity on Mental and Physical Health Outcomes in Older Adults With Arthritis." *Frontiers in Pain Research* 3 (2022): 886985. https://doi.org/10.3389/fpain.2022.886985.

Volpi, E., R. Nazemi, and S. Fujita. 2004. "Muscle Tissue Changes With Aging." *Current Opinion Clinical Nutrition and Metabolism Care* 7 (4): 405-410. https://doi.org/10.1097/01.mco.0000134362.76653.b2.

Warburton, D.E., C.W. Nicol, and S.S. Bredin. 2006. "Health Benefits of Physical Activity: The Evidence." *Canadian Medical Association Journal* 174 (6): 801-9. https://doi.org10.1503/cmaj.051351.

Xu, J., S.L. Murphy, K.D., Kochanek, and E. Arias. 2022. "Mortality in the United States, 2021." www.cdc.gov/nchs/products/databriefs/db456.htm.

CHAPTER 2

Buckinx, F., and M. Aubertin-Leheudre. 2019. "Menopause and High-Intensity Interval Training: Effects on Body Composition and Physical Performance." *Menopause* 26 (11): 1232-1233.

Grosicki, G.J., C.S. Zepeda, and C.W. Sundberg. 2022. "Single Muscle Fibre Contractile Function With Ageing." *Journal of Physiology* 600 (23): 5005-5026.

Schuenke, M.D., R.P. Mikat, and J.M. McBride. 2002. "Effect of an Acute Period of Resistance Exercise on Excess Post-Exercise Oxygen Consumption: Implications for Body Mass Management." *European Journal of Applied Physiology* 86 (5): 411-417.

Tremblay, A., J.A. Simoneau, and C. Bouchard. 1994. "Impact of Exercise Intensity on Body Fatness and Skeletal Muscle Metabolism." *Metabolism* 43 (7): 814-818.

Wewege, M., R. van den Berg, R.E. Ward, and A. Keech. 2017. "The Effects of High-Intensity Interval Training vs. Moderate-Intensity Continuous Training on Body Composition in Overweight and Obese Adults: A Systematic Review and Meta-Analysis." *Obesity Reviews* 18 (6): 635-646.

CHAPTER 3

Calder, P.C. 2010. "Omega-3 Fatty Acids and Inflammatory Processes." *Nutrients* 2 (3): 355-374.

Caron-Jobin, M., A.S. Morisset, A. Tremblay, C. Huot, D. Légaré, and A. Tchernof. 2011. "Elevated Serum 25(OH)D concentrations, Vitamin D, and Calcium Intakes Are Associated With Reduced Adipocyte Size in Women." *Obesity (Silver Spring)* 19 (7): 1335-1341.

Centers for Disease Control, Division of Nutrition, Physical Activity, and Obesity, National Center for Chronic Disease Prevention and Health Promotion. 2022. "Get the Facts: Data and Research on Water Consumption." www.cdc.gov/nutrition/data-statistics/plain-water-the-healthier-choice.html.

Chae, M., and K. Park. 2021. "Association Between Dietary Omega-3 Fatty Acid Intake and Depression in Postmenopausal Women." *Nutrition Research and Practice* 15 (4): 468-478.

Clear, J. 2018. *Atomic Habits*. New York: Penguin Random House.

Cleveland Clinic. 2021. "Cortisol." https://my.clevelandclinic.org/health/articles/22187-cortisol.

Covassin, N., P. Singh, S.K. McCrady-Spitzer, E.K. St. Louis, A.D. Calvin, J.A. Levine, and V.K. Somers. 2022. "Effects of Experimental Sleep Restriction on Energy Intake, Energy Expenditure, and Visceral Obesity." *Journal of American College of Cardiology* 79 (13): 1254-1265.

Davis, S.R., C. Castelo-Branco, P. Chedraui, M.A. Lumsden, R.E. Nappi, D. Shah, and P. Villaseca. 2012. "Understanding Weight Gain at Menopause." *Climacteric* 15 (5): 419-429.

Ekholm, B., S. Spulber, and M. Adler. 2020. "A Randomized Controlled Study of Weighted Chain Blankets for Insomnia in Psychiatric Disorders." *Journal of Clinical Sleep Medicine* 16 (9): 1567-1577.

Farshchi, H.R., M.A. Taylor, and I.A. Macdonald. 2004. "Decreased Thermic Effect of Food After an Irregular Compared With a Regular Meal Pattern in Healthy Lean Women." *International Journal of Obesity and Related Metabolic Disorders* 28 (5): 653-660.

Grigolon, R.B., G. Ceolin, Y. Deng, A. Bambokian, E. Koning, J. Fabe, M. Lima, F. Gerchman, C.N. Soares, E. Brietzke, and F.A. Gomes. 2023. "Effects of Nutritional Interventions on the Severity of Depressive and Anxiety Symptoms of Women in the Menopausal Transition and Menopause: A Systematic Review, Meta-Analysis, and Meta-Regression." *Menopause* 30 (1): 95-107.

Halton, T.L., and F.B. Hu. 2004. "The Effects of High-Protein Diets on Thermogenesis, Satiety and Weight Loss: A Critical Review." *Journal of the American College of Nutrition* 23 (5): 373-385.

Haskell, C.F., B. Robertson, E. Jones, J. Forster, R. Jones, A. Wilde, S. Maggini, and D.O. Kennedy. 2010. "Effects of a Multi-Vitamin/Mineral Supplement on Cognitive Function and Fatigue During Extended Multi-Tasking." *Human Psychopharmacology* 25 (6): 448-461.

Iwao, S., K. Mori, and Y. Sato. 1996. "Effects of Meal Frequency on Body Composition During Weight Control in Boxers." *Scandinavian Journal of Medicine & Science in Sports* 6 (5): 265-272.

Lerchbaum, E. 2014. "Vitamin D and Menopause: A Narrative Review." *Maturitas* 79 (1): 3-7. https://doi.org/10.1016/j.maturitas.2014.06.003.

Louis-Sylvestre, J., A. Lluch, F. Neant, and J.E. Blundell. 2003. "Highlighting the Positive Impact of Increasing Feeding Frequency on Metabolism and Weight Management." *Forum of Nutrition* 56: 126-128.

Maleki, S.J., J.F. Crespo, and B. Cabanillas. 2019. "Anti-Inflammatory Effects of Flavonoids." *Food Chemistry* 299: 125124.

Mettler, S., N. Mitchell, and K.D. Tipton. 2010. "Increased Protein Intake Reduces Lean Body Mass Loss During Weight Loss in Athletes." *Medicine and Science in Sports and Exercise* 42 (2): 326-337.

Mohammady, M., L. Janani, S. Jahanfar, and M.S. Mousavi. 2018. "Effect of Omega-3 Supplements on Vasomotor Symptoms in Menopausal Women: A Systematic Review and Meta-Analysis." *European Journal of Obstetrics, Gynecology, and Reproductive Biology* 228: 295-302.

Phillips, S.M., and L.J. Van Loon. 2011. "Dietary Protein for Athletes: From Requirements to Optimum Adaptation." *Journal of Sports Science* 29 (Suppl 1): S29-38.

Pietilä, J., E. Helander, I. Korhonen, T. Myllymäki, U.M. Kujala, and H. Lindholm. 2018. "Acute Effect of Alcohol Intake on Cardiovascular Autonomic Regulation During the First Hours of Sleep in a Large Real-World Sample of Finnish Employees: Observational Study." *JMIR Mental Health* 5 (1): e23.

Rosenblum, J.L., V.M. Castro, C.E. Moore, and L.M. Kaplan. 2012. "Calcium and Vitamin D Supplementation Is Associated With Decreased Abdominal Visceral Adipose Tissue in Overweight and Obese Adults." *The American Journal of Clinical Nutrition* 95 (1): 101-108.

Schwingl, P.J., B.S. Hulka, and S.D. Harlow. 1994. "Risk Factors for Menopausal Hot Flashes." *Obstetrics and Gynecology* 84 (1): 29-34.

Seo, J.A., H. Cho, C.R. Eun, H.J. Yoo, S.G. Kim, K.M. Choi, S.H. Baik, D.S. Choi, M.H. Park, C. Han, and N.H. Kim. 2012. "Association Between Visceral Obesity and Sarcopenia and Vitamin D Deficiency in Older Koreans: The Ansan Geriatric Study." *Journal of the American Geriatrics Society* 60 (4): 700-706.

Silva, T.R., K. Oppermann, F.M. Reis, and P.M. Spritzer. 2021. "Nutrition in Menopausal Women: A Narrative Review." *Nutrients* 13 (7): 2149.

Skoczek-Rubińska, A., A. Muzsik-Kazimierska, A. Chmurzynska, P.J. Walkowiak, and J. Bajerska. 2021. "Snacking May Improve Dietary Fiber Density and Is Associated With a Lower Body Mass Index in Postmenopausal Women." *Nutrition* 83: 111063.

Solianik, R., and A. Sujeta. 2018. "Two-Day Fasting Evokes Stress, But Does Not Affect Mood, Brain Activity, Cognitive, Psychomotor, and Motor Performance in Overweight Women." *Behavioural Brain Research* 338: 166-172.

Stokes, T., A.J. Hector, R.W. Morton, C. McGlory, and S.M. Phillips. 2018. "Recent Perspectives Regarding the Role of Dietary Protein for the Promotion of Muscle Hypertrophy With Resistance Exercise Training." *Nutrients* 10 (2): 180.

Varady, K.A., S. Cienfuegos, M. Ezpeleta, and K. Gabel. 2021. "Cardiometabolic Benefits of Intermittent Fasting." *Annual Review of Nutrition* 41: 333-361.

Wiley, T.S., and B. Formby. 2000. *Lights Out.* New York: Simon & Schuster.

CHAPTER 4

Haidt, J. 2006. *The Happiness Hypothesis: Finding Modern Truth in Ancient Wisdom.* New York: Basic Books.

Heath, C., and D. Heath. 2010. *Switch: How to Change Things When Change Is Hard.* New York: Broadway.

Hladek, M., J.M. Gill, C. Lai, K. Bandeen-Roche, Q.L. Xue, J. Allen, C. Leyden, R. Kanefsky, and S.L. Szanton. 2022. "High Social Coping Self-Efficacy Associated With Lower Sweat Interleukin-6 in Older Adults With Chronic Illness." *Journal of Applied Gerontology* 41 (2): 581-589.

Kite, L., and L. Kite. 2020. *More Than a Body: Your Body Is an Instrument, Not an Ornament.* New York: Harper Collins.

Teixeira, P.J., E.V. Carraça, D. Markland, M.N. Silva, and R.M. Ryan. 2012. "Exercise, Physical Activity, and Self-Determination Theory: A Systematic Review." *The International Journal of Behavioral Nutrition and Physical Activity* 9: 78.

CHAPTER 6

Bird, S.P., K.M. Tarpenning, and F.E. Marino. 2006. "Effects of Liquid Carbohydrate/Essential Amino Acid Ingestion on acute Hormonal Response During a Single Bout of Resistance Exercise in Untrained Men." *Nutrition* 22 (4): 367-375. https://doi.org/10.1016/j.nut.2005.11.005.

Brooks, J.D., W.E. Ward, J.E. Lewis, J. Hilditch, L. Nickell, E. Wong, and L.U. Thompson. 2004. "Supplementation With Flaxseed Alters Estrogen Metabolism in Postmenopausal Women to a Greater Extent Than Does Supplementation With an Equal Amount of Soy." *The American Journal of Clinical Nutrition* 79 (2): 318-325.

Ciloglu, F., I. Peker, A. Pehlivan, K. Karacabey, N. Ilhan, O. Saygin, and R. Ozmerdivenli. 2005. "Exercise Intensity and Its Effects on Thyroid Hormones." *Neuro Endocrinology Letters* 26 (6):830-834.

Cinar, V., Y. Polat, A.K. Baltaci, and R. Mogulkoc. 2011. "Effects of Magnesium Supplementation on Testosterone Levels of Athletes and Sedentary Subjects at Rest and After Exhaustion." *Biological Trace Element Research* 140 (1): 18-23.

Epel, E.S., B. McEwen, T. Seeman, K. Matthews, G. Castellazzo, K.D. Brownell, J. Bell, and J.R. Ickovics. 2000. "Stress and Body Shape: Stress-Induced Cortisol Secretion Is Consistently Greater Among Women With Central Fat." *Psychosomatic Medicine* 62 (5): 623-632.

Ingram, D.M., F.C. Bennett, D. Willcox, and N. de Klerk. 1987. "Effect of Low-Fat Diet on Female Sex Hormone Levels." *Journal of the National Cancer Institute* 79 (6): 1225-1229.

Janssen, I., L.H. Powell, R. Kazlauskaite, and S.A. Dugan. 2010. "Testosterone and Visceral Fat in Midlife Women: The Study of Women's Health Across the Nation (SWAN) Fat Patterning Study." *Obesity (Silver Spring)* 18 (3): 604-610.

Kraemer, W.J., N.A. Ratamess, W.C. Hymer, B.C. Nindl, and M.S. Fragala. 2020. "Growth Hormone(s), Testosterone, Insulin-Like Growth Factors, and Cortisol: Roles and Integration for Cellular Development and Growth With Exercise." *Frontiers in Endocrinology* 11: 33.

Lee, A.S.D. 2020. "The Role of Vitamin B6 in Women's Health." *The Nursing Clinics of North America* 56 (1): 23-32. https://doi.org/10.1016/j.cnur.10.002.

Masjedi, F., S. Keshtgar, F. Agah, and N. Karbalaei. 2019. "Association Between Sex Steroids and Oxidative Status With Vitamin D Levels in Follicular Fluid of Non-Obese PCOS and Healthy Women." *Journal of Reproduction & Infertility* 20 (3): 132-142.

Otun, J., A. Sahebkar, L. Östlundh, S.L. Atkin, and T. Sathyapalan. 2019. "Systematic Review and Meta-Analysis on the Effect of Soy on Thyroid Function." *Scientific Reports* 9 (1): 3964.

Sachmechi, I., A. Khalid, S.I. Awan, Z.R. Malik, and M. Sharifzadeh. 2018. "Autoimmune Thyroiditis With Hypothyroidism Induced by Sugar Substitutes." *Cureus* 10 (9): e3268.

Walter, K.N., E.J. Corwin, J. Ulbrecht, L.M. Demers, J.M. Bennett, C.A. Whetzel, and L.C. Klein. 2012. "Elevated Thyroid Stimulating Hormone Is Associated With Elevated Cortisol in Healthy Young Men and Women." *Thyroid Research* 5 (1):13. https://doi.org/10.1186/1756-6614-5-13.

Ward, L.J., S. Nilsson, M. Hammar, L. Lindh-Åstrand, E. Berin, H. Lindblom, A.C. Spetz Holm, M. Rubér, and W. Li. 2020. "Resistance Training Decreases Plasma Levels of Adipokines in Postmenopausal Women." *Scientific Reports* 10 (1): 19837.

Wideman, L., J.Y. Weltman, M.L. Hartman, J.D. Veldhuis, and A. Weltman. 2002. "Growth Hormone Release During Acute and Chronic Aerobic and Resistance Exercise: Recent Findings." *Sports Medicine* 32 (15): 987-1004. https://doi.org/10.2165/00007256-200232150-00003.

Yang, C.Z., S.I. Yaniger, V.C. Jordan, D.J. Klein, and G.D. Bittner. 2011. "Most Plastic Products Release Estrogenic Chemicals: A Potential Health Problem That Can Be Solved." *Environmental Health Perspectives* 119 (7): 989-996.

CHAPTER 7

Burke, L.E., J. Wang, and M.A. Sevick. 2011. "Self-Monitoring in Weight Loss: A Systematic Review of the Literature." *Journal of the American Dietetic Association* 111 (1):92-102. https://doi.org/10.1016/j.jada.2010.10.008.

Gallagher, D., S.B. Heymsfield, M. Heo, S.A. Jebb, P.R. Murgatroyd, and Y. Sakamoto. 2000. "Healthy Percentage Body Fat Ranges: An Approach for Developing Guidelines Based on Body Mass Index." *The American Journal of Clinical Nutrition* 72 (3): 694-701. https://doi.org/10.1093/ajcn/72.3.694.

Linde, J.A., R.W. Jeffery, S.A. French, N.P. Pronk, and R.G. Boyle. 2005. "Self-Weighing in Weight Gain Prevention and Weight Loss Trials." *Annals of Behavioral Medicine* 30 (3): 210-6. https://doi.org/10.1207/s15324796abm3003_5.

VanWormer, J.J., S.A. French, M.A. Pereira, and E.M. Welsh. 2008. "The Impact of Regular Self-Weighing on Weight Management: A Systematic Literature Review." *The International Journal of Behavioral Nutrition and Physical Activity* 5: 54. https://doi.org/10.1186/1479-5868-5-54.

Welsh, E.M., N.E. Sherwood, J.J. VanWormer, A.M. Hotop, and R.W. Jeffery. 2009. "Is Frequent Self-Weighing Associated With Poorer Body Satisfaction? Findings From a Phone-Based Weight Loss Trial." *Journal of Nutrition Education and Behavior* 41 (6): 425-428. https://doi.org/10.1016/j.jneb.2009.04.006.

CHAPTER 13

"The Female ACL: Why Is It More Prone to Injury?" 2016. *Journal of Orthopaedics* 13 (2): A1-A4. https://doi.org/10.1016/S0972-978X(16)00023-4.

Hunter, G.R., C.S. Bickel, G. Fisher, W.H. Neumeier, and J.P. McCarthy. 2013. "Combined Aerobic and Strength Training and Energy Expenditure in Older Women." *Medicine and Science in Sports and Exercise* 45 (7): 1386-1393.

ABOUT THE AUTHOR

Rachel Cosgrove, CSCS, has been the co-owner of Results Fitness with her husband, Alwyn Cosgrove, for over 20 years. Located in Southern California, it was voted one of the top 10 gyms in the United States by *Men's Health* magazine for three years in a row.

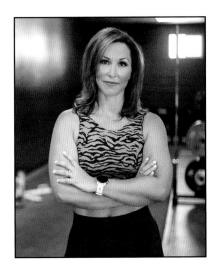

Cosgrove earned her bachelor's degree in physiology, with an emphasis on exercise and health, from the University of California–Santa Barbara. She holds the Certified Strength and Conditioning Specialist (CSCS) credential from the National Strength and Conditioning Association (NSCA) and is certified as a U.S. Olympic weightlifting coach and as a U.S. triathlon coach. She taught the very first USA Obstacle Course Racing Level 1 certification course at the U.S. Olympic Training Center in 2019. In addition to being one of the first people certified by the International Society of Sports Nutrition (ISSN), she has the Nutrition and Lifestyle Coach certification from the prestigious CHEK Institute and Precision Nutrition. She also holds the Russian Kettlebell certification, the Ultimate Sandbag certification, and the Functional Movement Screen certification.

Named IDEA Personal Trainer of the Year (2012), Cosgrove has been a featured expert in a number of magazines, including *Women's Health*, *Muscle and Fitness Hers*, *Oxygen*, *Shape*, *Men's Health*, *More*, *Real Simple*, *Women's World*, *U.S. News & World Report*, and *Men's Fitness*. She has also appeared on Fox, WGN, ABC, NBC, and the Dr. Oz show, and she was a spokesperson for Secret deodorant. She is a sought-after presenter at national and international conferences and events. She is the author of *The Female Body Breakthrough* and the *Women's Health*–branded book *Drop Two Sizes*. She has also served on the advisory board for *Women's Health* and Livestrong.com and worked as a consultant for Nike.

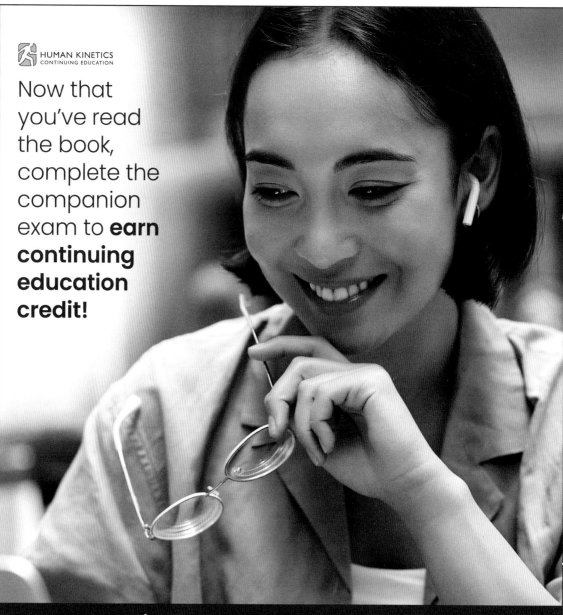
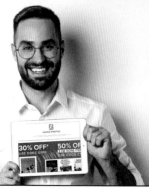